Common Diseases
Diseases
of Companion
Animals

Common Diseases *of* Companion Animals

ALLEICE SUMMERS, MS, DVM

Professor, Veterinary Technology
Cedar Valley College, Lancaster, Texas

with 89 illustrations

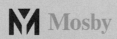 Mosby

An Affiliate of Elsevier Science
St. Louis   London   Philadelphia   Sydney   Toronto

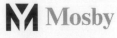

An Affiliate of Elsevier Science

Editorial Manager: Linda L. Duncan
Senior Developmental Editor: Teri Merchant
Project Manager: Linda McKinley
Senior Production Editor: Jennifer Furey
Design Coordinator: Julia Ramirez

Copyright © 2002 by Mosby, Inc.

NOTICE
Pharmacology is an ever-changing field. Standard safety precautions must be followed, but as new research and clinical experience broaden our knowledge, changes in treatment and drug therapy may become necessary or appropriate. Readers are advised to check the most current product information provided by the manufacturer of each drug to be administered to verify the recommended dose, the method and duration of administration, and contraindications. It is the responsibility of the treating veterinarian, relying on experience and knowledge of the patient, to determine dosages and the best treatment for each individual patient. Neither the Publisher nor the editor assumes any liability for any injury and/or damage to persons or property arising from this publication.

Permission to photocopy or reproduce solely for internal or personal use is permitted for libraries or other users registered with the Copyright Clearance Center, provided that the base fee of $4.00 per chapter plus $.10 per page is paid directly to the Copyright Clearance Center, 222 Rosewood Drive, Danvers, Massachusetts 01923. This consent does not extend to other kinds of copying, such as copying for general distribution, for advertising or promotional purposes, for creating new collected works, or for resale.

Mosby Inc.
An Affiliate of Elsevier Science
11830 Westline Industrial Drive
St. Louis, Missouri 63146

Printed in the United States of America

Library of Congress Cataloging in Publication Data

Summers, Alleice
    Common diseases of companion animals / Alleice Summers
        p. cm.
    Includes bibliographical references (p.)
    ISBN 0-323-01260-4
    1. Dogs—Diseases.   2. Cats—Diseases.   I. Title.

SF991 .S878 2002
636.7'0896—dc21

2001044528

02   03   04   05   06   GW/MV   9   8   7   6   5   4   3   2

To my parents
Clark and Margaret Toldan
who always believed I could succeed at whatever I attempted

To my students,
past and present,
whose questions inspired this book

PREFACE

Veterinary technicians serve a wide variety of functions in the clinical setting. Although they are not diagnosticians, they do assist the veterinarian, through assessment and laboratory procedures, in arriving at a diagnosis. Perhaps their most important functions are in treatment planning/implementation and client/patient follow-up and compliance. To perform these duties effectively, they need a strong understanding of diseases.

While teaching a course on small animal diseases for veterinary technology students at Fairmont State College, I discovered there was no text written expressly for the veterinary technician that covered this material. I realized that a handy reference was needed that offered a description of the most common diseases encountered in a small animal practice, including clinical signs, diagnostic tests and laboratory work, treatment, prevention, and client information. Just as important, this book seeks to delineate the role of the technician in all phases of diagnosis, treatment, and client communication.

Common Diseases of Companion Animals is a collection of both clinical and practical information concerning diseases seen frequently in the small animal practice. Tech Alerts are included throughout the text to emphasize the role of the technician in the total care of the patient. This book is written as a text for veterinary technology students and as a reference for daily clinical practice. It is not intended to be a comprehensive medical text; rather, the goal of this work is to acquaint veterinary technicians with disease processes and their treatments so that they may better educate their clients.

ORGANIZATION

The thirteen chapters of this book are organized according to organ system. In each chapter, specific diseases affecting each system follow an introductory section. Included in each section are clinical signs, suggested diagnostic texts, treatments, and information for clients. The client information section is designed to help the technician discuss the disease, treatment, and prevention with the client. The book is written in a easy-to-read style, with clinical signs, diagnostic tests, and treatments displayed in a monograph form for easy reference. Because this book is a reference, students are often asked to review anatomy, physiology, surgery, and clinical pathology texts and other works for additional information. It is hoped that the information presented in this book will partner with the education provided to the technician by the veterinarian to provide the technician a fuller appreciation of the disease processes seen in small animals.

ACKNOWLEDGMENTS

I would like to thank my colleagues who so generously gave their time to make suggestions for improvements to this book. I would also like to acknowledge my co-workers Brian Heim, Marge Haney, Bill Lineberry, Vicki Van Huss, Mark Wilson, Charles Wolf, and David Wright, who supported my work by providing a great working environment that allowed me the freedom to pursue this project. Also, thanks to Candy Tooley, Teri Sweet, and Sandra Smith for helping select the illustrations. Last but not least, I would like to thank all my clients and their wonderful pets who, over the last 21 years, have provided me with many laughs, tears, and experiences that I will never forget.

ALLEICE SUMMERS

CONTENTS

Common
Diseases
of Companion
Animals

The Body Defense Systems—The Body's Response to Disease

one

Animals, as well as their owners, live their lives in an unfriendly, hostile environment. They are continually assaulted by hordes of microorganisms such as bacteria, viruses, protozoans, fungi, and parasites. Internally, abnormal cells produced by cellular division must continually be removed from the body. If allowed to survive, they become tumors. Some of these tumors may become malignant, spreading throughout the body. Tissues within the body are continually being repaired or replaced as they wear out or become damaged. With all this activity going on in the body, it is a wonder that animals and humans survive this environment.

IMMUNITY

The body has developed an efficient system of defense against disease-producing agents—the *immune system*. Components of this system patrol the body 24 hours a day looking for foreign and internal enemies. The activities of this system are called *immunity;* without it, animals could not survive. Immunity can be divided into two large categories: nonspecific immunity and specific immunity.

NONSPECIFIC IMMUNITY

Nonspecific immunity is comprised of several elements: species resistance, mechanical and chemical barriers, the inflammatory response, interferon, and

1

complement. The term *nonspecific* means that the system responds to all antigenic insults in the same manner, not specifically to any one type of pathogenic organism.

SPECIES RESISTANCE

Species resistance refers to the genetic ability of a particular species to provide defense against certain pathogens. For example, canines do not get feline leukemia virus, and felines do not contract canine distemper virus. Neither species can contract plant diseases. A knowledge of species resistance can allow a clinician or veterinary technician to focus on the group of diseases seen in that animal species and not spend time ruling out those that do not appear.

MECHANICAL AND CHEMICAL BARRIERS

The animal's internal body is protected by a mechanical barrier, the skin and the mucous membranes. If unbroken, this barrier prevents the entry of microorganisms, protecting the underlying tissues from injury. The skin also produces substances such as sebum, mucus, and enzymes that act to inhibit or destroy pathogens. Damage to this barrier allows organisms to reach the internal structures of the body and produce disease. Healthy skin is the animal's best defense against the world of microorganisms. It is called the "first line of defense."

INFLAMMATORY RESPONSE

If bacteria or other invaders do gain access to the body, a "second line of defense," known as the *inflammatory response,* exists. When a tissue is invaded by microorganisms or injured in any way, the cells that make up that tissue release enzymes called *mediators,* which attract white blood cells to the area *(chemotaxis),* dilate blood vessels, and increase the permeability of the vessels in the area. The characteristic signs of inflammation—heat, redness, swelling, and pain—occur as a result of the release of these chemical substances. Specific types of white blood cells (usually neutrophils) attracted to the area will begin to "gobble up" the invading foreign material in a process known as *phagocytosis.* The increased blood flow to the area will increase the temperature of the tissue, inhibiting the growth of new organisms. It also brings in raw materials for the repair of the damaged tissue and clotting factors to assist in hemorrhage control. With time, the body is able to clean up the damage and return the tissue to its normal state.

INTERFERON AND COMPLEMENT

Chemicals produced by cells invaded by viruses also make up part of nonspecific immunity. Interferon is a substance that interferes with the ability of viruses to cause disease by preventing their replication within the host cell. Complement, another group of enzymes, is activated during infections. Complement binds to the invading cell wall, producing small holes in the membrane. This results in rupture, or *lysis,* of the foreign cell.

SPECIFIC IMMUNITY

Specific immunity, the "third line of defense," is carried out by two types of white blood cells called *lymphocytes.* There are two main categories of lymphocytes, *B-cell lymphocytes* and *T-cell lymphocytes.* B-cell lymphocytes produce antibodies in response to specific *antigen* stimulation. This is known as the *humoral response.* T-cell lymphocytes interact more directly with the pathogens by combining directly with the foreign cell and destroying it or rendering it incapable of causing disease. Because this response is more direct than that of the B cell, it is known as *cell-mediated immunity.*

CELL-MEDIATED IMMUNITY

T cells originate in the bone marrow of the animal. After leaving the bone marrow and entering the circulation, they arrive at the *thymus,* a glandular structure found in the mediastinum just cranial to the heart. The thymus is the primary central gland of the lymphoid system and is very large in young animals but decreases in size as the animal matures. Here the T cells "go to college," where they are programmed to recognize the markers that are unique on the cells of that specific individual *(self-recognition).* After "graduation," the T cells move out into the spleen and lymph nodes and circulate through the body, constantly on the lookout for invading substances.

Macrophages, a type of white blood cell, also travel through the tissues looking for foreign substances. When they find one, they attach to it and take the invader to the T cell. The T cell then attaches to the receptor site on the invading cell and divides repeatedly. All the new T cells then migrate to the site of the infection and begin to destroy the invading organisms. T-cell response is rapid and deadly to pathogens.

HUMORAL IMMUNITY

B-cell response (humoral) is a slower type of immune response. Like T cells, B cells originate within the animal's bone marrow or in the bursa of Fabricius in

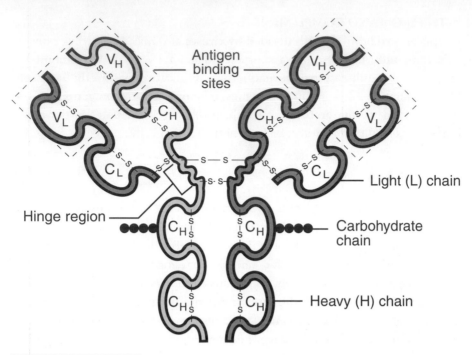

FIGURE 1-1. Chemical structure of the immunoglobulin G (IgG) class of antibody. Each molecule is composed of four polypeptide chains (two heavy and two light) plus a short carbohydrate chain attached to each heavy chain. The variable chain gives the immunoglobulin its specificity. V, Variable region; C, constant region; V_L, variable region of light chain; C_L, constant region of light chain; V_H, variable region of heavy chain; C_H, constant region of heavy chain; s-s, sulfur-sulfur bonds.

some species. Young, inactive B cells produce *antigen-combining receptor sites* over the surface of their cell membranes. Upon contact with a specific antigen, the cell divides repeatedly, producing a *clone* of identical B cells. Some of these B cells become *plasma cells* and are stimulated to produce large protein molecules called *antibodies*. Others remain as *memory cells,* which have the ability to recognize the antigen if it is ever again presented to them. Each clone of B cells, and hence each antibody, is specific for only one antigen. The antibody produced is a large protein molecule *(immunoglobulin)* whose chemical structure contains an area able to lock onto the antigen (Fig. 1-1). Combining with the antigen may result in rendering the antigen harmless to the body, may cause antigens to clump together *(agglutinate)* and be removed from solution, or may result in the destruction of the antigenic cell. This humoral response is not immediate. It takes time for the B cells to clone and begin to produce antibodies. Within 7 to 10 days after the initial infection, antibodies can be found in the body. However, if the animal has been exposed to the antigen previously and memory cells are present, this time period is shorter.

B-cell and T-cell immunity can be further classified according to the manner in which they develop. *Inherited immunity* occurs as a result of genetic factors that influence the developing fetus before birth. *Acquired immunity* is resistance that develops after the animal is born. Acquired immunity may be either *natural* or *artificial*. Natural immunity occurs every time the animal is exposed to a pathogen. It is a continual process in the animal world. Artificial immunity is usually the result of a deliberate exposure to a pathogen such as with vaccinations. Both natural and artificial immunity can be further divided into either *passive* or *active immunity*. In passive immunity, antibodies formed in one infected animal are transferred to another animal that is not infected. This, then, provides the uninfected animal with protection against the pathogen. Active immunity occurs when the animal's own immune system encounters a pathogen and responds by producing an immune response.

The ultimate result of both specific and nonspecific immunity is that the body eliminates foreign substances, whether they are bacteria, viruses, protozoa, parasites, or the body's own cells gone bad. If this system fails or is overwhelmed, disease occurs. Many factors affect the proper functioning of the immune system, such as nutrition, stress, sanitation, and age. Concurrent disease can also weaken the immune system, allowing other organisms to gain access to the body. Veterinary technicians must be familiar with the effect these elements have on the health of the animals in their care and be able to educate pet owners in the areas necessary for the healthy life of their pets.

WHAT HAPPENS WHEN THE SYSTEM DOES NOT FUNCTION PROPERLY?

The following chapters of this book discuss some of the most commonly seen diseases of domestic animals. The technician should keep the function of the immune system in mind as these diseases are discussed. When the function of the immune system is disrupted, animals become ill.

THE CARDIOVASCULAR SYSTEM two

The cardiovascular system plays an important role in maintaining homeostasis throughout the body. It performs this function by regulating the flow of blood through miles of vessels and capillaries. It is in the capillaries that vital nutrient transport into the body cells and removal of waste materials from the cells occurs.

To understand cardiovascular disease, one must first study the anatomy and physiology of the cardiovascular system. (The student is referred to an anatomy and physiology text for a detailed description.) Simply stated, the system is one composed of a pump (the heart) and pipes (the vessels). The heart circulates fluid (blood) through the vessels where it delivers its content to the cells and removes waste products (Fig. 2-1). This system is a "closed" system—change in one portion of the system affects the other portions of the system.

ANATOMY AND PHYSIOLOGY

THE HEART

At the center of this system is the heart, a four-chamber pump designed to rhythmically contract, pumping blood to all parts of the body. Specialized cardiac muscle cells located in the sinoatrial (SA) node generate electrical impulses that spread over the heart through a specialized conduction system, resulting in simultaneous contraction of the cardiac muscle cells. This contraction pushes blood *into* the arterial vessels and returns blood to the heart from the veins. Using an *electrocardiograph* (ECG), the clinician can measure this electrical activity as it moves across the surface of the body (Fig. 2-2). The ECG

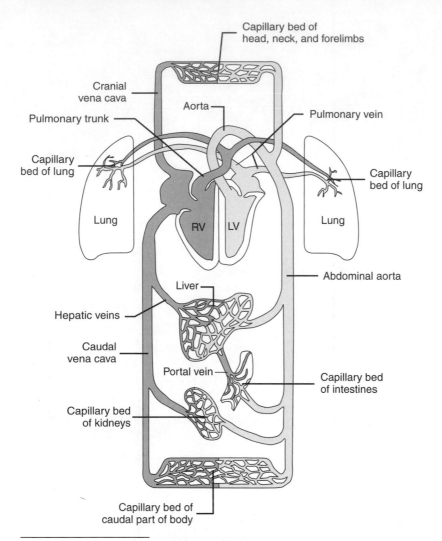

Capillary bed of
head, neck, and forelimbs

Cranial
vena cava

Aorta

Pulmonary trunk

Pulmonary vein

Capillary
bed of lung

Capillary
bed of lung

Lung

RV LV

Lung

Abdominal aorta

Liver

Hepatic veins

Caudal
vena cava

Portal vein

Capillary bed
of intestines

Capillary bed
of kidneys

Capillary bed of
caudal part of body

FIGURE 2-1. Systemic and pulmonary circulation. *LV,* Left ventricle; *RV,* right ventricle. (From Colville T, Bassert JM: *Clinical anatomy and physiology for veterinary technicians,* St Louis, 2002, Mosby.)

measures the electrical activity generated by the heart by the placement of electrodes at specific points on the body surface. Each mechanical contraction of the heart is preceded by an electrical wave front that stimulates heart muscle contraction. This electrical wave front begins at the SA node and travels to the muscle cells of the ventricle through the cardiac conduction system. These

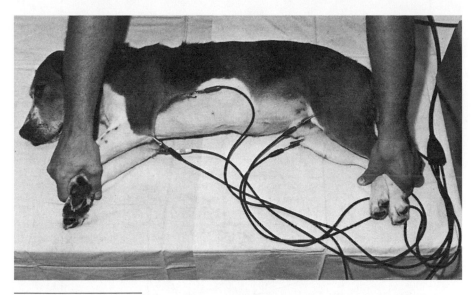

FIGURE 2-2.   Using an electrocardiograph. (From Edwards NJ: *Bolton's handbook of canine and feline electrocardiography,* ed 2, Philadelphia, 1987, WB Saunders.)

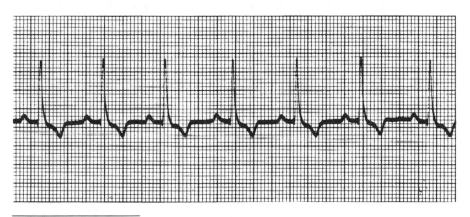

FIGURE 2-3.   Normal electrocardiogram of a dog. (From Edwards NJ: *ECG manual for the veterinary technician,* Philadelphia, 1993, WB Saunders.)

wave fronts are recorded as an electrocardiogram. Fig. 2-3 shows a normal electrocardiogram of a dog. Fig. 2-4 represents the normal pathway for electrical conduction through the heart.

The electrical activity of this pump is automatic but can be adjusted by input from the *neuroendocrine system* to meet the demands of the animal's body.

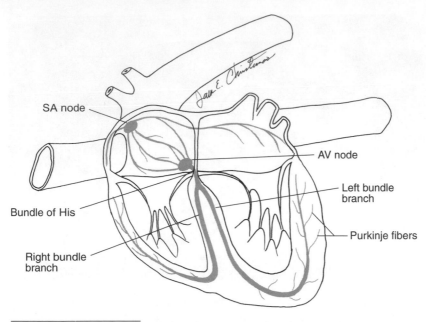

Figure 2-4. Normal pathway for electrical conduction through the heart. (From McBride DF: *Learning veterinary terminology,* ed 2, St Louis, 2002, Mosby.)

Many cardiac diseases involve a failure of this pump to function properly. *Congestive heart failure, cardiomyopathy, valvular disease,* and *congenital malformations* can all affect the pumping efficiency of the heart and ultimately the function of the entire body.

The Vessels

Connected to the pump are a series of vessels. Arteries carry oxygenated blood at high pressure (the systolic blood pressure) to arterioles and on to capillaries where exchange of nutrients and gases occurs. Blood then moves into venules, through veins, and is returned to the right side of the heart. Arteries are capable of dilation and constriction, routing blood to areas where it is needed and away from those areas not in need. Constriction serves to increase blood pressure and dilation serves to decrease it.

Vascular diseases affect the flow of blood through the body and, ultimately, its return to the heart. If the volume of blood returning to the heart is abnormal, the heart will compensate by altering the rate of contraction, the strength of contraction, or both, to return homeostasis to the circulatory system.

HEART FAILURE

When the blood returning to the heart cannot be pumped out at a rate matching the body's need, *heart failure* occurs. There are many causes of heart failure and the disease is often difficult to explain. The clinical signs of the disease and treatment regimens depend on *individual* patient diagnosis and evaluation. The veterinarian must determine whether the failure is the result of myocardial dysfunction (pump failure) or circulatory failure (lack of circulating fluid volume).

Myocardial dysfunction is seen in diseases such as the following:

- Cardiomyopathy
- Myocarditis
- Taurine deficiency (cats)
  Circulatory failure results from the following:
- Hypovolemia (shock, hemorrhage, dehydration)
- Anemia
- Valvular dysfunction
- Congenital shunts or defects

Heart failure is termed *congestive heart failure* when the failing heart allows fluid congestion to accumulate in the body, resulting in edema. Most heart failure will become "congestive" as the pump progressively fails.

CARDIOMYOPATHIES

CANINE DILATED CARDIOMYOPATHY (DCM)

DCM is one of the most common acquired cardiovascular diseases of dogs. It is primarily a disease of older, male, large and giant breed dogs such as Scottish Deerhounds, Dobermans, Boxers, Irish wolfhounds, Saint Bernards, Newfoundlands, Afghans, and Old English Sheepdogs. The disease has also been seen in English and American Cocker Spaniels. It is rare in dogs weighing less than 12 kg.

The pathology of the disease involves dilation of all chambers of the heart. This dilation (due to weak, thin, and flabby cardiac muscle) results in a decreased cardiac output and an increase in cardiac afterload (blood left in the heart during diastole). The etiology of this disease is unknown, although viral, nutritional, immune-mediated, and genetic causes have been proposed. DCM results in impaired systolic function of the ventricles and, therefore, decreased stroke volume (the volume of blood ejected from the heart with each contraction). The effect on the animal is one of low-output circulatory failure, exhibited by weakness, exercise intolerance, syncope, or shock.

Dogs with DCM frequently develop atrial fibrillation, which further contributes to a decrease in cardiac output. Signs of atrial fibrillation include rapid, irregular heart rhythms and sudden death.

CLINICAL SIGNS
- Right heart failure: ascites, hepatomegaly, weight loss, abdominal distension
- Left heart failure: coughing, pulmonary edema, syncope
- Exercise intolerance

DIAGNOSIS
- Radiographs may show an enlarged heart in some dogs.
- Ultrasonography indicates chambers dilated and other signs consistent with DCM.
- ECG shows widened QRS and P waves and rhythm disturbances.

TREATMENT
- There is no cure. Treatment is aimed at keeping the dog comfortable.
- Diuretics: furosemide 1.1 to 2 mg/kg q 8 to 12 h
- Digoxin: 0.01 to 0.02 mg/kg PO b.i.d. Monitor digoxin blood levels (1 to 2 ng/ml)
- Enalapril: 0.5 mg/kg q 12 h

INFORMATION FOR CLIENTS
- This is almost always a fatal disease.
- Most dogs will die within 6 months to 2 years.
- Dogs may die suddenly from malignant cardiac arrhythmia.
- The disease appears to be more prevalent in certain breeds of dogs.

CANINE HYPERTROPHIC CARDIOMYOPATHY (HCM)

In this uncommon disease of dogs, the left ventricular muscle hypertrophies, decreasing the filling capacity of the ventricle and often blocking the outflow of blood during systole. The etiology appears to be heritable.

CLINICAL SIGNS
- Fatigue
- Cough

- Tachypnea
- Syncope
- Presence or absence of cardiac murmurs
- Sudden death
- Some animals may be asymptomatic.

DIAGNOSIS
- Ultrasonography indicates concentric thickening and hypertrophy of the left ventricle.

TREATMENT
- None routinely used

INFORMATION FOR CLIENTS
- Sudden death and congestive heart failure may occur in dogs with HCM.
- The disease may run in families of certain breeds: German Shepherds, Rottweilers, Dalmatians, Cocker Spaniels, Boston Terriers, Shih Tzu.

FELINE DILATED CARDIOMYOPATHY

Before the late 1980s, feline dilated cardiomyopathy was one of the most frequent cardiac diseases reported in cats. After the association of the disease with taurine deficiency, additional taurine was added to commercial diets, and the incidence of the disease significantly decreased. The pathology is similar to DCM in dogs. There is evidence of a genetic predisposition to DCM in cats fed taurine-deficient diets.

CLINICAL SIGNS
- Dyspnea
- Inactivity
- Anorexia
- Acute lameness or paralysis, usually in the rear limbs
- Pain and lack of circulation in the affected limbs
- Hypothermia

DIAGNOSIS
- Clinical signs
- ECG shows increased QRS voltages, wide P waves, ventricular arrhythmia.
- Ultrasonography shows dilated heart chambers.

TREATMENT

- Oral taurine supplementation: 250 to 500 mg/day
- Furosemide: 0.55 to 2.2 mg/kg q 8 to 24 h
- Oxygen
- Digoxin: 0.005 to 0.008 mg/kg/day PO b.i.d.
- Enalapril: 0.25 to 0.5 mg/kg PO s.i.d. to b.i.d.
- Cutaneous nitroglycerin paste: ¼ inch q 8 to 12 h
- Hydralazine: 0.44 to 0.88 mg/kg q 12 h PO

❶ TECH ALERT

Avoid IV fluid replacement in cats until pulmonary edema or pulmonary effusion is under control.

INFORMATION FOR CLIENTS

- The most critical period is the first 2 weeks of treatment.
- Cats that survive the first 2 weeks of treatment and that do well on taurine supplementation have a good prognosis. Cats that do not respond to taurine have a poor long-term prognosis.

❶ TECH ALERT

Be extremely careful when handling these cats. Affected cats can die suddenly while you are attempting to collect laboratory samples or obtain radiographs.

FELINE HYPERTROPHIC CARDIOMYOPATHY

HCM in cats is similar to the disease in dogs; left ventricular hypertrophy is the predominant pathology. Neutered, male cats between the ages of 1 and 16 years of age have been found to be most at risk. The etiology of the disease may be related to abnormal myocardial myosin or calcium transport within the muscles of the heart.

CLINICAL SIGNS

- Soft, systolic murmur (grade 2 to 3/6)
- Gallop rhythms or other arrhythmia
- Acute onset of heart failure or systemic thromboembolism

DIAGNOSIS

- Radiographs may show a normal size heart or mild left atrial enlargement.
- ECG shows increased P wave duration, increased QRS width, and sinus tachycardia.
- Ultrasound shows increased left ventricular wall thickness and a dilated left atrium.

TREATMENT

- Furosemide: 6.25 to 12.5 mg q 8 to 12 h PO
- Propranolol: *cats <4.5 kg,* 2.5 mg b.i.d. to t.i.d. PO; *cats >5 kg,* 5 mg b.i.d. to t.i.d. PO, *or* diltiazem 0.5 to 2.5 mg/kg q 8 h PO
- Monitor ECG/heart rate, blood pressure; may see bradycardia and hypotension at the higher doses

INFORMATION FOR CLIENTS

- Cats with HCM may experience heart failure, arterial embolism, and sudden death.
- Cats with heart rates <200 beats/min have a better prognosis than cats whose rates are >200 beats/min.
- The median survival time is about 732 days.

THROMBOEMBOLISM

Thrombus formation is a common and serious complication of myocardial disease in the cat. It is estimated that between 10% and 20% of cats with HCM will develop thrombi in the left heart, which may dislodge and become trapped elsewhere in the arterial system. Cats seem to have inherently high platelet reactivity, making clot formation a more likely sequel to endothelial damage and sluggish blood flow occurring with myocardial disease. Approximately 90% of these emboli lodge as "saddle thrombi" in the distal aortic trifurcation, resulting in hind limb pain and paresis. Rarely a thrombus will lodge at other arterial sites such as the renal artery, the coronary arteries, the cerebral arteries, or the mesenteric artery.

The goal of treatment is to dissolve the thrombus and restore perfusion to the area. Several drugs have been tried with varying results. Tissue plasminogen activator (TPA) has shown some success but is expensive. Heparin has also been used with some success. Low-dose aspirin therapy (22 mg/kg PO q 3 days) can be used prophylactically in cats with myocardial disease.

CLINICAL SIGNS
- Acute onset of rear leg pain and paresis
- Cold, bluish footpads (i.e., decreased circulation)
- Lack of palpable pulses in rear limbs
- History or clinical findings of myocardial disease

DIAGNOSIS
- Clinical signs
- Nonselective angiography if available

TREATMENT
- TPA (Activase, Genentech): give IV at a rate of 0.24 to 0.99 mg/kg/hr (to total IV dose of 10 mg/kg) *or* heparin: give IV 200 IU/kg followed by maintenance dose of 66 IU/kg q 6 h SQ.
- Prophylaxis: aspirin 22 mg/kg q 3 days

INFORMATION FOR CLIENTS
- Cats that develop painful, cold, or paralyzed rear legs should been seen at the hospital immediately.
- The prognosis for cats with thromboembolism is guarded to poor.
- Surgical removal of the thrombus is difficult.

CONGENITAL HEART DISEASE

Although malformations of the heart and great vessels represent a minor cause of clinical heart disease, it is important to identify them in newly acquired pets or those to be used for breeding. Technicians should be encouraged to use their stethoscopes to routinely listen to the heart. With practice, subtle changes will become noticeable, allowing the technician to note abnormalities in the patient's record.

Many malformations have a genetic basis. Breed predilections for congenital heart disease are listed in Table 2-1.

The diagnostic approach for congenital heart disease should include a good history, with special attention paid to breed, sex, and age of the patient. Clinical signs of congenital heart failure include failure to grow, dyspnea, weakness, syncope, cyanosis, seizures, and sudden death; however, many animals with congenital malformations may be asymptomatic.

TABLE 2-1. Canine breed predilections for congenital heart disease

BREED	DEFECT(s)
Basset Hound	PS
Beagle	PS
Bichon Frisé	PDA
Boxer	SAS, PS, ASD
Boykin Spaniel	PS
Bull Terrier	MVD, AS
Chihuahua	PDA, PS
Chow Chow	PS, CTD
Cocker Spaniel	PDA, PS
Collie	PDA
Doberman Pinscher	ASD
English Bulldog	PS, VSD, TOF
English Springer Spaniel	PDA, VSD
German Shepherd	SAS, PDA, TVD, MVD
German Shorthair Pointer	SAS
Golden Retriever	SAS, TVD, MVD
Great Dane	TVD, MVD, SAS
Keeshond	TOF, PDA
Labrador Retriever	TVD, PDA, PS
Maltese	PDA
Mastiff	PS, MVD
Newfoundland	SAS, MVD, PS
Pomeranian	PDA
Poodle	PDA
Rottweiler	SAS
Samoyed	PS, SAS, ASD
Schnauzer	PS
Shetland Sheepdog	PDA
Terrier breeds	PS
Weimaraner	TVD, PPDH
Welsh Corgi	PDA
West Highland White Terrier	PS, VSD
Yorkshire Terrier	PDA

From Sisson DD, Thomas WP, Bonagura JD: Congenital heart disease. In Ettinger SJ, Feldman EC: *Textbook of veterinary internal medicine,* ed 5, vol I, Philadelphia, 2000, WB Saunders.
AS, Aortic stenosis; *ASD,* atrial septal defect; *CTD,* cor triatriatum dexter; *MVD,* mitral valve dysplasia; *PDA,* patent ductus arteriosus; *PPDH,* peritoneopericardial diaphragmatic hernia; *PS,* pulmonic stenosis; *SAS,* subaortic stenosis; *TOF,* tetralogy of Fallot; *TVD,* tricuspid valve dysplasia; *VSD,* ventricular septal defect.

Most cases of congenital abnormalities are identified after the pet has been purchased, during the first visit to the veterinarian. On examination, a loud murmur often accompanied by a precordial trill may be heard. With some defects, the clinician may observe pulse abnormalities, cyanosis, jugular pulses, or abdominal distension. Laboratory tests may all be normal.

Although radiographs may suggest cardiac disease in some animals, echo-cardiography can provide an accurate diagnosis of the defect.

Causes of congenital heart disease include genetic, environmental, infectious, nutritional, and drug-related factors. More is understood of the genetic factors than the others. Studies suggest the defects are polygenic, and that they might be difficult to eliminate entirely from a specific breed.

This section will discuss the most commonly seen congenital defects. The student is referred to cardiology texts for a more detailed description of each defect.

Patent Ductus Arteriosus (PDA)

Failure of the ductus arteriosus to close following parturition results in blood shunting from the systemic circulation to the pulmonary artery. Normally the ductus carries blood from the pulmonary artery to the aorta during fetal development. The increase in oxygen tension in the blood at birth results in closure of the path in the first 12 to 14 hours of life. If the ductus remains open, blood will hyperperfuse the lung and the left side of the heart will become volume overloaded (Fig. 2-5). The resulting cardiac murmur is often referred to as a "machinery murmur" heard best over the main pulmonary artery high on the left base.

CLINICAL SIGNS
- Usually a female dog; Chihuahuas, Collies, Maltese, Poodles, Pomeranians, English Springers, Keeshonds, Bichon Frisés, and Shetland Sheepdogs are most commonly affected.
- Presence of loud murmur heard best over left thorax.
- Some puppies may be asymptomatic.

DIAGNOSIS
- Echocardiography reveals left ventricular dilation, aortic and pulmonary artery dilation.
- Radiographs show overcirculation of the pulmonary tree with left atrial and ventricular enlargement.

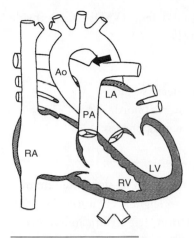

FIGURE 2-5.   Circulation in a dog with a large left-to-right shunting patent ductus arteriosus (PDA). The shunt results in pulmonary overcirculation and left ventricular volume overload. *RA,* Right atrium; *RV,* right ventricle; *LA,* left atrium; *LV,* left ventricle; *PA,* pulmonary artery; *Ao,* aorta. (From Kittleson MD, Kienle RD: *Small animal cardiovascular medicine,* St Louis, 1998, Mosby.)

TREATMENT
- Surgical correction should be accomplished before the age of 2 years.

INFORMATION FOR CLIENTS
- The prognosis is excellent with surgical correction.
- Without surgery, 64% of dogs with PDA will die within 1 year of diagnosis.
- Dogs with this condition should *not* be used for breeding.

ATRIAL AND VENTRICULAR SEPTAL DEFECTS

During fetal development, the atria and the ventricles are joined as a common chamber. The atria are partitioned by two septa and a slitlike opening (the foramen ovale) that allows right-to-left shunting of blood in the fetus. The ventricular septum is formed from several primordial areas. Eventually the atrial septum and the ventricular septum join in the area of the endocardial cushions. Defects in the structure of these septa result in patencies of the atrioventricular septum. This defect is fairly common in the cat. With atrial septal defects (ASDs), blood will typically shunt from left to right, overloading the right side of the heart. With ventricular septal defects (VSDs), the left side of the heart is usually overloaded and enlarged (Fig. 2-6).

CLINICAL SIGNS
- ASD: Soft, systolic murmur, split second heart sound
- VSD: Harsh, holosystolic murmur, right sternal border
- Signs of congestive heart failure before 8 weeks of age

DIAGNOSIS
- Radiographs reveal right heart enlargement with ASD, increased pulmonary vascularity, and left atrium normal to slightly enlarged. In VSD, radiographs reveal pulmonary overcirculation, left atrium and ventricle enlarged, and variable right ventricular enlargement.
- Echocardiography demonstrates the septal defect.

TREATMENT
- ASD: Medical management of congestive heart failure
- VSD: Medical management of congestive heart failure

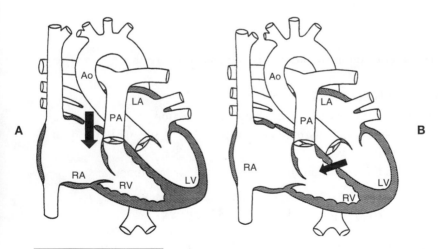

FIGURE 2-6.   A, Circulation in a dog with a large left-to-right shunting atrial septal defect (ASD). The shunt results in right ventricular volume overload (not shown) and pulmonary overcirculation. There is mild systolic pulmonary hypertension. B, Medium-size ventricular septal defect. The diameter of the defect is less than the diameter of the aorta, so it imposes resistance to blood flow. RA, Right atrium; RV, right ventricle; LA, left atrium; LV, left ventricle; PA, pulmonary artery; Ao, aorta. (From Kittleson MD, Kienle RD: Small animal cardiovascular medicine, St Louis, 1998, Mosby.)

INFORMATION FOR CLIENTS
- Repair of these defects requires open-heart surgery or cardiopulmonary bypass. This is uncommon in the dog or cat.
- Most of these animals will eventually develop congestive heart failure and require treatment.

STENOTIC VALVES (PULMONIC AND AORTIC VALVES)

Pulmonary stenosis results when the pulmonic valves are dysplastic or malformed. The lesion results in a narrowing of the outflow tract from the right ventricle. Obstruction to right ventricular outflow causes an increase in ventricular systolic pressure resulting in right ventricular hypertrophy. The right atrium also becomes enlarged. Severe stenosis limits cardiac output during exercise.

CLINICAL SIGNS
- Specific breeds (Chihuahua, Samoyed, English Bulldog, Miniature Schnauzer, Labrador Retriever, Mastiff, Chow Chow, Newfoundland, Basset Hound, terriers, and spaniels)
- Age greater than 1 year
- Syncope (fainting)
- Tiring on exercise
- Right-sided congestive heart disease
- Prominent jugular pulse
- Left basilar murmur
- Palpable right ventricular enlargement

DIAGNOSIS
- Radiographs reveal right ventricular enlargement, poststenotic dilation of the pulmonary artery, and pulmonary underperfusion.
- Echocardiography reveals right ventricular hypertrophy and enlargement, increased echogenicity of the pulmonary valves, and dilation of the main pulmonary artery.

TREATMENT
- Balloon valvuloplasty to relieve the obstruction
- Valvulotomy or partial valvulectomy to open the outflow tract
- Patch graft over the outflow tract to alleviate the obstruction
- Medical management of congestive heart failure

INFORMATION FOR CLIENTS

- Affected animals should not be used for breeding.
- Dogs with mild to moderate pulmonary stenosis can live normal lives.
- Sudden death may occur in dogs with moderate to severe pulmonary stenosis.

SUBAORTIC STENOSIS

This lesion occurs predominantly in large breed dogs. The Newfoundland, Boxer, German Shepherd, Golden Retriever, and Bull Terrier are the most commonly affected. In the Newfoundland, a genetic basis most compatible with an autosomal dominant mechanism has been proposed. The lesion develops during the first 4 to 8 weeks of life. The lesion consists of thickening of the endocardial tissue just below the aortic valve. The fibrous thickening results in obstruction to outflow, producing left ventricular hypertrophy, left atrial hypertrophy, and dilation of the aorta. Coronary artery circulation may also be affected. Severe subaortic stenosis (SAS) may lead to left-sided congestive heart failure or sudden death.

CLINICAL SIGNS

- Typical breed
- Soft to moderate ejection murmur of fourth left intercostal area
- Exertional tiring
- Syncope
- Left congestive heart failure
- Sudden death

DIAGNOSIS

- Radiographs reveal normal or left ventricular hypertrophy and widened mediastinum (from aortic dilation).
- Echocardiography reveals left ventricular hypertrophy, subvalvular fibrous ring, and poststenotic dilation of the aorta. In advanced stages, echocardiography may indicate left ventricular hypertrophy.

TREATMENT

- Exercise restriction
- Balloon catheter dilation of the stenotic ring
- Medical management: propranolol (for dogs with syncope and elevated pressure gradients), 0.55 to 1.1 mg/kg q 8 h

INFORMATION FOR CLIENTS

- These dogs should not be used for breeding.
- Most patients will develop left-sided congestive heart failure; the onset may be sudden.
- Sudden death is not uncommon in these dogs.
- Endocarditis (inflammation of the lining of the heart) is a risk in all cases of SAS.

TETRALOGY OF FALLOT

Tetralogy of Fallot is a polygenic, genetically transmitted malformation of the heart. Components include right ventricular outflow obstruction (pulmonary stenosis), secondary right ventricular hypertrophy, subaortic VSD, and overriding aorta (Fig. 2-7).

This condition is seen in the Keeshond, English Bulldog, and the cat. It occasionally occurs in other breeds of dogs. Symptoms may vary with the severity of the defects.

The presence of these malformations results in increased right-sided resistance and pressure and a right-to-left shunt between the pulmonary and

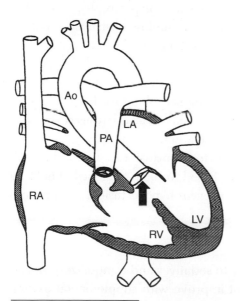

FIGURE 2-7. Circulation in a patient with tetralogy of Fallot with severe right ventricular outflow obstruction. Systolic pressures in the right ventricle *(RV)*, left ventricle *(LV)*, and aorta *(Ao)* are identical. (From Kittleson MD, Kienle RD: *Small animal cardiovascular medicine,* St Louis, 1998, Mosby.)

systemic circulations. Because of this pressure gradient, deoxygenated blood from the right ventricle shunts through the VSD to mix with oxygenated blood in the left ventricle. Blood flow to and from the pulmonary vasculature is minimal. This shunting results in hypoxemia, cyanosis, and secondary polycythemia. Right ventricular hypertrophy occurs. The murmur of pulmonary stenosis can usually be detected on the left hemithorax and, less often, a VSD murmur can be heard as well.

CLINICAL SIGNS
- Failure to grow
- Cyanosis
- Exercise intolerance, shortness of breath
- Weakness
- Syncope, seizures
- Sudden death

DIAGNOSIS
- Radiographs show a normal size heart and decreased pulmonary circulation.
- Echocardiography reveals right ventricular hypertrophy, small left chambers, large subaortic VSD, and right outflow obstruction. Bubble or Doppler studies indicate right-to-left shunting.

TREATMENT
- Surgical: Creation of a systemic to pulmonary shunt has been successful in increasing pulmonary circulation, venous return, left heart size, and oxygen saturation in the systemic circulation.
- Medical: Phlebotomy can be performed to maintain the packed cell volume between 62% and 68%. Blood volume removed should be replaced with crystalloid fluids to prevent hypoperfusion. Hypoxia can be treated with cage rest and oxygen.

● TECH ALERT
These animals may react adversely to sedatives and tranquilizers, developing a bradycardia that does not improve with supplemental oxygen therapy.

INFORMATION FOR CLIENTS
- This is a genetically transmitted disorder. These animals should not be used for breeding.

- Sudden death is common, but some animals can tolerate the defect for years.
- Congestive heart failure rarely develops from this disorder.
- Limit stress and exercise in these animals.
- Tranquilizers and sedatives may have an adverse effect on these animals.
- Regular phlebotomy (blood drawing) will be required to maintain a normal red blood cell level.

PERSISTENT RIGHT AORTIC ARCH AND OTHER VASCULAR RING ANOMALIES

Persistence of the right fourth aortic arch is a common malformation. The defect results in regurgitation of solid food in weanlings due to obstruction of the esophagus by the retained arch. It is a common defect in German Shepherds, Irish Setters, Great Danes, and is frequently seen in other large breeds.

CLINICAL SIGNS
- Regurgitation of solid food
- Aspiration pneumonia, fever, dyspnea, cough
- Weight loss

DIAGNOSIS
- Radiology: Barium swallow indicates constriction of the esophagus near the base of the heart. Solid food can be mixed with barium to establish constriction and retention of food in the esophagus.

TREATMENT
SURGICAL
- Surgery should be done early to obtain a better prognosis. This surgery is similar to surgery for PDA, because the ductus arteriosus is part of the vascular ring anomaly.

MAINTENANCE
- Feed semisolid or pelleted diet (frequent, small amounts).
- Feed from a height to avoid food build-up in the esophagus.
- Give antibiotics for respiratory infections.

INFORMATION FOR CLIENTS
- Without early surgical correction the prognosis is poor.
- Even with surgical correction some amount of esophageal dilation

will persist. This may result in vomiting if large boluses of food are consumed.

- These dogs should *not* be used for breeding.

ACQUIRED VALVULAR DISEASES

CHRONIC MITRAL VALVULAR INSUFFICIENCY (CMVI)

CMVI is the most commonly encountered cardiovascular disorder in the dog. The prevalence of this disease increases with age; as many as 75% of all dogs older than 16 years are affected. CMVI is rare in the cat. This disease is a progressive disorder, resulting in an estimated 95% of all cases of congestive heart failure in small-breed dogs.

The lesion consists of proliferation of fibroblastic tissue within the structure of the valve leaflets. This results in the nodular thickening of the valvular free edges, which then contract and roll up. The stiff, malformed leaflets fail to close sufficiently during systole, resulting in regurgitation of blood back up into the left atrium. The left atrium and, infrequently, the left ventricle dilate. The dilated atrium may result in pulmonary congestion and compression of the left mainstem bronchus, producing coughing and dyspnea.

One of the most common causes for mitral valvular insufficiency in older animals is chronic periodontal disease. Bacteria (mostly gram-negative anaerobes) living in tartar in periodontal pockets are showered into the bloodstream, colonizing the valve leaflets and resulting in their thickening. When the valve leaflets become inflamed and thickened, they fail to close properly, resulting in leakage of blood back into the left ventricle. The overload can then result in heart failure over time.

CLINICAL SIGNS

- Cough (deep, resonant, and usually worse at night or with exercise)
- Dyspnea, tachypnea
- Decreased appetite
- Systolic murmur, left apex; "whooping" quality

DIAGNOSIS

- Radiology: If pulmonary edema is present, venous engorgement will be present (vein diameter will be greater than that of the arteries). "Cotton-like" alveolar densities or air bronchograms will be present.

Without edema, left atrial and ventricular enlargement, elevation of the thoracic trachea, and loss of the "cardiac waist" can be seen on the lateral view. In the DV view, the enlarged left auricle can be seen as a bulge in the cardiac silhouette at the 2- to 3-o'clock position.

- Echocardiography reveals increased diameter of the left atrium and left ventricle. There is marked reduction in left ventricular contractility. The mitral valve leaflets may be thickened or prolapsed.

TREATMENT

- The main goal of treatment is to improve the length and the quality of life for the patient. No therapy will prolong survival or delay the start of treatment. Treatments are adjusted as the disease progresses, so varying combinations of medications may be used.

MEDICAL

- Diuretics to reduce the circulatory blood volume to the left side of the heart. Furosemide: initially 4.4 mg/kg q 8 to 12 h PO for 2 to 3 days followed by q 2 h for 3 to 7 days, then decreasing to 2.2 mg/kg q 24 h
- Arterial dilators to decrease systemic resistance. Hydralazine: initially 0.55 mg/kg PO q 12 h then increase in weekly intervals to 2.2 mg/kg PO q 12 h; enalapril: 0.27 to 0.55 mg/kg PO q 12 to 24 h
- Digoxin: 0.22 mg/m^2 PO q 12 h to keep heart rate below 160 beats/min in small dogs

INFORMATION FOR CLIENTS

- This is a progressive disease. Your pet will have to be reevaluated periodically and medications adjusted to provide him or her with adequate relief of symptoms.
- There is no cure for this condition.
- A low-salt diet such as Hills H/D will aid in preventing fluid accumulation in the body. Treats and table foods containing salt should be avoided.
- Eventually a point will be reached when medications do not relieve the clinical symptoms.

TRICUSPID VALVE INSUFFICIENCY

This disease is exactly like mitral valve insufficiency, but the signs are predominantly those of *right*-sided heart failure: pleural effusion, abdominal distension, hepatomegaly, and gastrointestinal signs such as vomiting, diarrhea, or anorexia. Treatment is basically the same as for mitral insufficiency. Repeated abdominocentesis is often required.

CARDIAC ARRHYTHMIAS

Arrhythmias may be defined as deviations from the normal heart rate or rhythm originating from abnormal locations within the heart. Many times no observable anatomic pathology in the myocardium that correlates with the rhythm disturbance exists.

Alterations in normal rhythm result from either *abnormal impulse formation* or *abnormal impulse conduction* within cardiac muscle fibers. (The student is referred to a physiology text to review nerve conduction and muscle contraction.) Altered impulse formation may occur as a result of ischemia (decreased supply of oxygenated blood), hypocalcemia (low calcium levels), cardiomyopathy, hypercalcemia (high calcium levels), excess catecholamines, or reperfusion injury. Conduction disturbances result when alternate pathways develop for repolarization of cardiac muscle.

Arrhythmias affect the hemodynamics of the body. Cerebral blood flow is reduced as much as 8% to 12% by premature beats, 14% by supraventricular (originating above the ventricles) tachycardias (rapid rates), 23% by atrial fibrillation, and 40% to 75% by ventricular tachycardia.

Many arrhythmias can be easily auscultated and confirmed by electrocardiogram. Treatment involves correcting the underlying cause, when possible, or controlling the arrhythmia when it is not possible to correct the underlying cause.

Supraventricular arrhythmias may be atrial (P wave positive but abnormal) or junctional (P wave negative in lead II). This class of arrhythmias includes the following:
- Supraventricular tachycardia
- Atrial premature contractions
- Atrial fibrillation

In supraventricular tachycardia (or sinus tachycardia), the heart rate typically exceeds 160 to 180 beats/min in the dog, although the P-QRS-T complexes remain normal. The heart rate may be slowed by vagal stimulation. Situations such as fear, excitement, exercise, anemia, or hyperthyroidism may cause this arrhythmia. The ECG displays normal complexes with a higher-than-normal heart rate (Fig. 2-8).

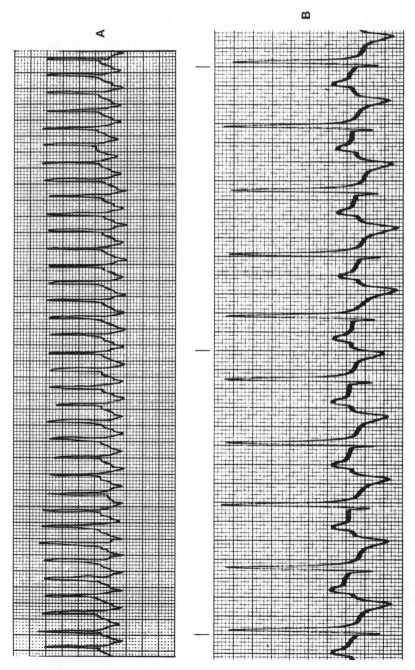

FIGURE 2-8. **A,** Atrial tachycardia. **B,** Supraventricular tachycardia. (**A,** From Edwards NJ: *ECG manual for the veterinary technician,* Philadelphia, 1993, WB Saunders; **B,** from Edwards NJ: *Bolton's handbook of canine and feline electrocardiography,* ed 2, Philadelphia, 1987, WB Saunders.)

In atrial premature contractions, abnormal P waves, occurring earlier than would normally be expected, are seen on the ECG. The P wave is usually followed by a normal QRS complex. These premature contractions may be associated with left atrial enlargement or atrial disease of any type (chronic mitral valve insufficiency). Animals are usually asymptomatic, but the technician may palpate a pulse deficit and auscultate a variable heart sound (Fig. 2-9). This arrhythmia may progress to atrial fibrillation.

ATRIAL FIBRILLATION (SUPRAVENTRICULAR ARRHYTHMIA)

Atrial fibrillation occurs when there is no organized atrial contraction. Cardiac output drops owing to the loss of atrial "kick" and the rapid ventricular rate. A critical mass of myocardial tissue is required to sustain atrial fibrillation; so the larger the heart, the more likely atrial fibrillation is to occur. Therefore it is more prevalent in large-breed dogs and dogs with cardiac diseases that increase the size of the heart (Fig. 2-10). *Ventricular arrhythmias* arise from the fibers of the ventricle. The QRS complexes are abnormally wide and bizarre, and they may or may not be related to the preceding P wave.

CLINICAL SIGNS
- Large-breed dog, with or without concurrent heart disease
- Weakness, syncope
- Collapse
- Rapid, irregular heart rate

DIAGNOSIS
- Auscultation of a rapid, irregular heart rate
- ECG: no evidence of P waves, irregular base line; rapid, irregular rate

TREATMENT
- Treatment aims to slow the heart rate; treatment will not correct the atrial fibrillation.
- Digitalis glycosides to slow rate—Digoxin: 0.22 mg/m² PO b.i.d. for dogs; cats: 0.005 to 0.008 mg/kg/day PO b.i.d.
- Calcium channel blockers to slow AV node conduction and increase the refractory period:
     Diltiazem: 0.4 to 1.5 mg/kg PO q 8 h for dogs; 0.5 to 1 mg/kg PO q 8 h for cats
     Verapamil: 1.1 to 4.4 mg/kg PO q 8 to 12 h (dogs only)

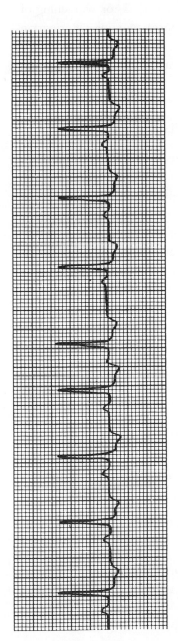

Figure 2-9. Atrial premature contractions. (From Edwards NJ: *ECG manual for the veterinary technician*, Philadelphia, 1993, WB Saunders.)

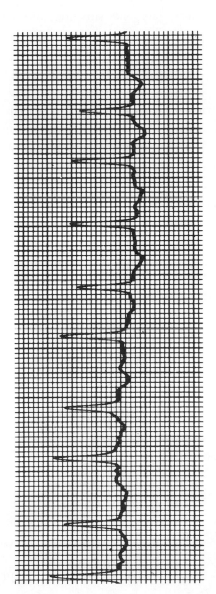

Figure 2-10. Atrial fibrillation. (From Edwards NJ: *Bolton's handbook of canine and feline electrocardiography*, ed 2, Philadelphia, 1987, WB Saunders.)

INFORMATION FOR CLIENTS
- Treatment will not cure the atrial fibrillation.
- Concurrent heart disease will progress even with treatment.
- Congestive heart failure will eventually develop.
- Periodic examinations and reevaluations of the pet will be necessary.
- Report any gastrointestinal upset, anorexia, diarrhea, or worsening of cardiac function (coughing, weakness, collapse) to your veterinarian immediately.
- In an emergency situation, inform the person treating your pet about the drugs your pet has been taking.

VENTRICULAR TACHYCARDIA (VENTRICULAR ARRHYTHMIA)

Ventricular tachycardia may be associated with diseases such as cardiomyopathy, congestive heart failure, endocarditis or myocarditis, or cardiac neoplasia. Electrolyte and acid-base imbalances will also produce ventricular tachycardia. The rapid rate of contraction reduces ventricular filling time and, therefore, decreases cardiac output. If allowed to progress, ventricular tachycardia may lead to ventricular fibrillation, a life-threatening condition. Ventricular fibrillation is equivalent to cardiac arrest because no blood is moved into the systemic circulation due to inadequate myocardial contractions and poor filling of the ventricles (Fig. 2-11).

CLINICAL SIGNS
- Weakness, collapse, and syncope with rapid ventricular rates
- Sudden death in many cases
- Congestive heart failure with long-standing ventricular tachycardias

DIAGNOSIS
- Auscultation
- ECG: Infrequent to frequent widened, bizarre QRS complexes of ventricular origin. In ventricular fibrillation, abnormal baseline with no QRS complexes.

TREATMENT
- Treat if the number of ventricular premature contractions (VPCs) is >25/min, heart rate is >130 beats/min, the breed is at risk for sudden death, or clinical symptoms exist.
- Procainamide: 6.6 to 22 mg/kg PO q 4 h (dogs)

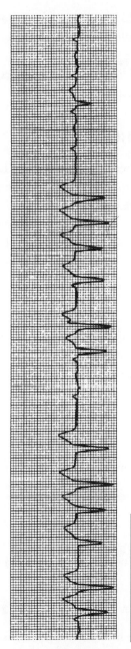

FIGURE 2-11. Ventricular tachycardia. (From Edwards NJ: *ECG manual for the veterinary technician*, Philadelphia, 1993, WB Saunders.)

- Tocainide: 5 mg/kg PO q 8 to 12 h (dogs)
- Lidocaine (2% without epinephrine): 4.4 to 8 mg/kg IV **slow** bolus. If ventricular fibrillation: cardiac defibrillation, IV fluids, sodium bicarbonate; all based on standard cardiopulmonary resuscitation techniques.

INFORMATION FOR CLIENTS
- Prognosis is guarded unless the underlying cause of the arrhythmia can be resolved.
- German Shepherds and Boxers are breeds that experience sudden death from ventricular tachycardia.

VENTRICULAR FIBRILLATION

In ventricular fibrillation, there is a complete lack of well-defined QRS complexes—a lack of heart sounds, blood pressure, and pulse (Fig. 2-12). Ventricular fibrillation is a life-threatening condition that must be corrected immediately with intubation and respiratory assist, IV fluid therapy, cardiac massage, epinephrine, and possibly electric defibrillation.

SINUS ARRHYTHMIA

Sinus arrhythmia is a common, normal occurrence in dogs. It is related to breathing and alterations in vagal tone that occur during inspiration and expiration. Heart rates increase during inspiration and decrease during expiration (Fig. 2-13). If one listens carefully, this arrhythmia can be heard in almost every dog examined. It is not seen in cats.

SINUS BRADYCARDIA

Sinus bradycardia is also a commonly seen arrhythmia, especially in large-breed dogs and athletic, highly conditioned animals. The electrocardiogram shows normal P and QRS complexes with a rate less than 70 beats/min. Pathologic conditions that may produce this arrhythmia include increased intracranial pressure, hyperkalemia (excess potassium), hypothyroidism, gastrointestinal disturbances, drugs, or any condition that results in increased vagal tone (neck trauma, tumors, etc.).

CLINICAL SIGNS
- Usually none unless the heart rate drops drastically
- Episodic weakness, syncope, collapse

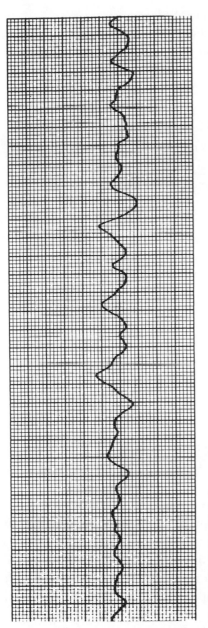

FIGURE 2-12. Ventricular fibrillation. (From Edwards NJ: *ECG manual for the veterinary technician,* Philadelphia, 1993, WB Saunders.)

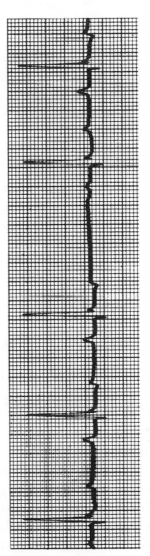

FIGURE 2-13. Sinus arrhythmia. (From Edwards NJ: *Bolton's handbook of canine and feline electrocardiography,* ed 2, Philadelphia, 1987, WB Saunders.)

DIAGNOSIS
- Auscultation
- ECG: slow rate with normal P, QRS complexes

TREATMENT
- None unless clinical signs are present
- Atropine: 0.02 to 0.04 mg/kg IV or IM (dogs, cats)
- Propantheline: 0.5 to 1.0 mg/kg PO t.i.d. (dogs); 0.8 to 1.6 mg/kg t.i.d. (cats), but usually ineffective
- Placement of pacemaker

INFORMATION FOR CLIENTS
- This may be a normal finding in athletic dogs.
- Correction of concurrent problems may eliminate the bradycardia.
- Most dogs can live a normal life with this disorder, but if clinical symptoms of weakness or syncope develop, treatment may be necessary.

❶ TECH ALERT
Brachiocephalic dogs and cats can develop severe bradycardias during intubation. It is important to carefully monitor the patient and avoid traumatic techniques that overstretch the neck or traumatize the vagus nerve.

HEARTWORM DISEASE

CANINE HEARTWORM DISEASE

Heartworm disease is of worldwide significance. In the United States, the disease is concentrated in areas within 150 miles of the coastal regions from Texas to New Jersey and along the Mississippi River and its tributaries, but can be seen anywhere due to the tremendous mobility of the canine population. The disease is spread by many different species of mosquitoes. Male dogs are more frequently infected than females (4:1), and outside dogs are more likely to become infected than inside dogs. Infections are normally detected between 3 and 8 years of age. Large-breed dogs appear to be more susceptible to infection than small breeds, and cats appear to be resistant to the disease. (Mosquito bites are less common in cats.)

The female mosquito serves as the intermediate host by obtaining a blood meal containing the microfilaria of *Dirofilaria immitis* from an infected dog. These microfilaria develop in the mosquito within 2 to 2.5 weeks and are then injected into the skin of another dog through a bite. The infective larvae migrate within the skin of the new host for about 100 days. Young adults (L5 stage) enter the vasculature and migrate to the pulmonary artery where they mature into adults. Approximately 6 months after the initial bite, microfilaria can be detected in the blood of the host dog.

Disease severity is partially related to the number of adult heartworms. The presence of adult worms in the pulmonary artery damages the endothelial lining of the vessel and increases the permeability, allowing fluid and proteins to leak into the perivascular tissue. The *physical* presence of the parasites results in right-sided heart enlargement (blockage of the right outflow tract) and pulmonary hypertension.

Heartworm disease is easily detected using immunodiagnostic tests that use monoclonal antibodies against heartworm uterine antigen. Microfilaria can be detected using filter techniques, the Knott's test, or by simply observing a drop of whole blood under the microscope, although these methods may miss as many as 25% of infected dogs.

Treatment involves the removal of the adult worms by the use of thiacetarsamide (Caparsolate, Rhone-Merieux) or melarsamine dihydrochloride (Immiticide, Merial) followed by a microfilaricide (ivermectin). Animals are then placed on daily or monthly prophylaxis.

CLINICAL SIGNS
Most dogs are asymptomatic, and infections are discovered on routine screening during yearly examinations. Clinical signs include the following:
- Cough, dyspnea
- Exercise intolerance
- Hemoptysis (coughing up blood)
- Signs of right heart failure

DIAGNOSIS
- Positive antigen test
- Positive concentration test
- Radiographs show evidence of pulmonary changes consistent with heartworm disease—right ventricular enlargement, increased prominence of pulmonary artery, enlarged lobar arteries, and increased perivascular pattern.

TREATMENT

If treatment is elected, the animal should have a pretreatment laboratory workup, which includes a minimum of a CBC, serum chemistries, and chest radiographs.

Adulticide treatment

- Thiacetarsamide: Given as 4 IV injections over a period of 2 days. Dose is 2.2 mg/kg b.i.d. for 2 days.
  1. Use of a butterfly catheter is recommended. Extravasation into perivascular tissues *will* result in a severe tissue sloughing.
  2. Use a different site for each injection.
- Melarsamine dihydrochloride: 2.6 mg/kg IM given at 24-hour intervals. Injections should be made deep into the lumbar muscle.
- Both of these drugs are toxic. Signs of toxicity may occur during or after treatment.
  1. Thiacetarsamide: Toxicity occurs in approximately 10% to 15% of cases. Signs include bilirubinuria, vomiting, anorexia, lethargy, and icterus.
  2. Melarsamine hydrochloride: Signs of toxicity include respiratory distress, vomiting, panting, excessive salivation, and diarrhea.

Treatment of toxicities

- Thiacetarsamide: stop treatment; give IV balanced electrolyte solutions; feed high-carbohydrate, low-fat diet; and limit exercise.
- Melarsamine dihydrochloride: dimercaprol (British anti-Lewisite in oil).

Microfilaricide treatment

- Give 3 to 6 weeks after the adulticide treatment.
- Ivermectin: 0.048 mg/kg given as a single dose (dilute 1 ml of Ivomec or Equavalen with 9 ml of propylene glycol or water and dose at 0.05 ml/kg)
- Milbemycin oxime: 0.48 mg/kg given as a single dose

❶ TECH ALERT

Use care in treating collies because they have a genetic susceptibility to ivermectin toxicity.

PREVENTION

- Diethylcarbamazine (DEC): Given daily at dose of 1.1 to 1.3 mg/kg

⚠ TECH ALERT
Do not use DEC in heartworm-positive dogs.

- Ivermectin: 5.98 µg/kg given monthly
- Milbemycin oxime: 0.51 mg/kg monthly

FELINE HEARTWORM DISEASE

In areas where heartworm disease is prevalent, cats are also at risk of infection. Until recently, it has been difficult to diagnose the disease in cats because they are usually negative for microfilaria, and the canine heartworm antigen tests are inadequate for detecting the disease in cats.

Cats are resistant to *Dirofilaria immitis* infection, having few adult worms, which are eliminated from the host within 2 years. Outside male cats are most at risk of infection. The mean age of diagnosis is between 3 and 6 years.

Symptoms in cats differ from those in dogs. Sudden death of an asymptomatic cat is fairly frequent. Most symptoms relate to the respiratory system (cough, dyspnea) or the gastrointestinal tract (vomiting, anorexia, lethargy). Acute pulmonary embolism occurs with affected cats demonstrating severe dyspnea, weakness, and anorexia. Ataxia, blindness, and seizures can also be seen.

Prevention is advised and is now available for cats at risk. Treatment regimens are controversial. In most cases, treatment involves supportive care while the cat eliminates the parasite.

CLINICAL SIGNS
- Coughing, dyspnea
- Vomiting
- Anorexia, weight loss
- Lethargy
- Right-sided congestive heart failure
- Sudden death or acute development of neurologic signs

DIAGNOSIS
- Feline heartworm antibody immunodiagnostic tests (can be done in-house)
- Radiographs: Signs are similar to those in the canine but are more difficult to interpret.

❶ TECH ALERT

Use caution when radiographing dyspneic cats—undue restraint may kill the cat!

- ECG should be performed in all cases. Check for adult worms in the pulmonary artery.

TREATMENT

Adulticide treatment is usually *not* recommended in the cat. However, if treatment is prescribed:

- Thiacetarsamide: 2.2 mg/kg IV q 12 h for 2 days (more effective in dogs)

❶ TECH ALERT

Most treated cats (half to two thirds) will develop signs of toxicity—depression, anorexia, and vomiting. Pulmonary edema is common post-treatment.

- Microfilaricide is not needed in cats (lack of microfilaria).
- Cage rest
- Cortisone may be used to decrease the inflammatory component of the disease.
- Prevention: milbemycin oxime 0.5 to 0.99 mg/kg PO monthly; *or* ivermectin 0.024 mg/kg PO q 30 to 45 days

Diseases of the Digestive System

three

Food is vital for the life of the animal because it provides the source of energy that drives all the chemical reactions in the body. Consumed food is not in a form readily useable by the body. The digestive system breaks down the consumed food to a point where it can be absorbed and used by the animal.

The organs of digestion can be divided into two main groups, the gastrointestinal tract, a continuous tube beginning at the mouth and ending at the anus, and the *accessory structures:* the teeth, tongue, salivary glands, liver, pancreas, and gallbladder (Fig. 3-1).

A discussion of diseases affecting the gastrointestinal system can best be approached by dividing the system into regions: oral cavity and esophagus, stomach, small bowel, large bowel, liver, pancreas, and rectum and anus.

ORAL DISEASES

Diseases of the oral cavity most frequently seen in small animals include the following: gingivitis/periodontal disease, lip-fold dermatitis, trauma, salivary mucocele, and oral neoplasms. Clinical signs for these diseases are similar; the animals are reluctant to eat and have oral pain, halitosis, and excessive salivation.

GINGIVITIS/PERIODONTAL DISEASE

Periodontal disease results from infectious inflammation of the gingiva and affects all the structures involved with tooth attachment (Fig. 3-2). This condition is a continuum of disease beginning with gingivitis and progressing to periodontitis and tooth loss. *Gingivitis*, a reversible process involving inflammation

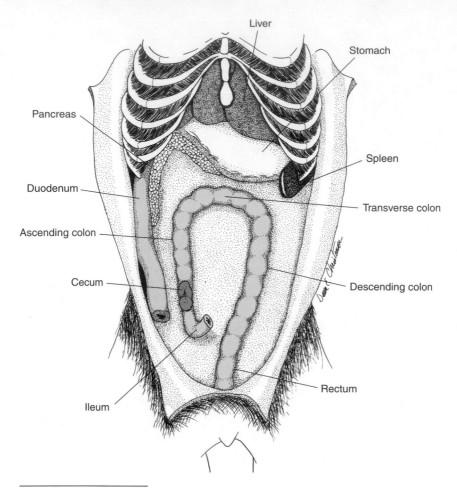

FIGURE 3-1.   Gastrointestinal system of dog (small intestine has been removed). (From Christenson DE: *Veterinary medical terminology,* Philadelphia, 1997, WB Saunders.)

of the margins of the gums, is caused by accumulation of tartar on the teeth, which acts as a nidus for bacterial multiplication. Enzymes produced by these bacteria damage the tooth attachments and result in inflammation. Without intervention, gingivitis will progress to *periodontitis,* an irreversible condition resulting in loss of gingival epithelial root attachment and alveolar bone reabsorption. Periodontal disease is estimated to occur in 60% to 80% of dogs and cats.

CLINICAL SIGNS
- Halitosis
- Reluctance to chew hard food, bones, toys
- Pawing at the mouth

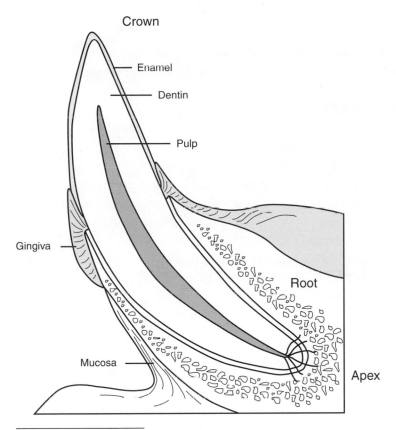

FIGURE 3-2.   Cross-section of a typical tooth. (From Colville T, Bassert JM: *Clinical anatomy and physiology for veterinary technicians,* St Louis, 2002, Mosby.)

- Head shyness
- Oral pain
- Personality changes
- Sneezing, nasal discharge
- Increased salivation (may be bloody)
- Facial swelling
- Tooth loss

DIAGNOSIS

- Complete oral examination (may require general anesthesia or sedation)
- Increased depth of the gingival sulcus (dogs >3 mm; cats >1 mm)
- Presence of tartar on the teeth, inflammation

TREATMENT
- Dental scaling, extraction of all loose teeth
- Root planing
- Gingival curettage
- Sublingual lavage
- Antibiotics (clindamycin, enrofloxacin, clavamox)
- Instruct owners in developing a good oral hygiene program.

INFORMATION FOR CLIENTS
- Good oral hygiene is a necessity for all pets. It should begin around 2 years of age or when needed.
- Brush teeth daily to remove tartar and plaque.
- Have routine dental cleanings performed by your veterinarian.
- Treat gingivitis early, before the development of irreversible signs.
- Some animals may require extraction of all their teeth to remove the source of infection.
- Hard, crunchy foods may promote better dental health by manually removing tarter before it calcifies. Once calcified, tartar must be removed professionally.

LIP-FOLD DERMATITIS

Lip-fold dermatitis is commonly seen in breeds with pendulous upper lips and prominent lower lip folds. Breeds such as spaniels, setters, bulldogs, and bassets are most commonly affected. Constant moisture of these folds from saliva results in increased bacterial growth. Along with the collection of food and hair in the area, the saliva causes increased irritation, erythema, and a fetid odor.

CLINICAL SIGNS
- Halitosis
- Collection of debris in the lower lip folds

DIAGNOSIS
- Clinical signs, especially in breeds predisposed to problems with lip folds
- Complete blood work to rule out other causes of halitosis and lip-fold disease such as periodontal disease, *Demodex* infestation, pemphigus, and renal failure

TREATMENT

- Complete dental cleaning
- Flush and clean lip folds with 2.5% benzoyl peroxide shampoo.
- Surgical resection of lip folds may be required in some cases.

INFORMATION FOR CLIENTS

- Keep the lip folds clean and dry.
- Daily cleaning will be required for the life of the animal.
- Drying agents such as cornstarch may help some animals. Dust them into the folds several times daily after cleaning.
- Good dental hygiene will benefit these animals.

ORAL TRAUMA

Oral trauma is common in small animals. Falls, fights, burns, blunt trauma, penetration of foreign objects, and automobile accidents account for many injuries to the oral cavity of pets. Head injuries from "high-rise syndrome" (e.g., cats falling from windows of buildings) or from other types of accidents often result in fracture of the mandibular symphysis, maxillary dysfunction, and/or separation of the hard palate of cats. The tongue is frequently injured by self-trauma (biting its own tongue), dog fights, penetration of foreign bodies (e.g., splinters, needles, bullets), or strangulation by elastic or stringlike materials. Cats that play with needles and thread may injure the tongue or frenulum or have a linear foreign body lodged somewhere in the oral cavity. Tongue lacerations have occurred as a result of dogs and cats attempting to eat from discarded tin cans to which the lids are still attached.

Electrical and chemical burns are often seen in young, curious animals that cannot resist biting an electric cord or tasting unusual plants or liquids. Electrical burns not only involve the mucosal surface of the oral cavity, but progress deep into the tissue along vessels and wet tissue planes. Contact with caustic chemicals and plants can result in erosion of the oral mucosa, producing pain, inflammation, secondary infection, and necrosis.

Gunshot wounds often result in dental or other oral injuries as well as shattered bones, teeth, and penetrating wounds of the tongue.

Fishhooks of all types attract both dogs and cats. Hooks can become embedded in the lips or the tongue (sometimes both at the same time), resulting in a frantic animal that may require sedation or general anesthesia to properly remove the hook.

Round steak bones present a special challenge. These bones typically become lodged behind the canine teeth, over the end of the mandible. As the tissue swells, it becomes painful. General anesthesia is required in most cases. Bones must be cut in sections for removal. Cats also have problems with bones; flat chicken bones can become lodged across the upper dental arcade, requiring sedation for removal.

CLINICAL SIGNS

- History or signs of head trauma
- Increased salivation
- Inability to close the mouth
- Reluctance or inability to eat
- Presence of a foreign body

DIAGNOSIS

- Physical examination of the oral cavity
- Radiographs to rule out the presence of an embedded linear foreign body

TREATMENT

- Treatment depends on the extent of the damage.
- Control bleeding.
- Provide supportive treatment: fluids, pain relief.
- Maintain an adequate airway.
- Perform lavage with copious amount of water in the case of chemical burns.
- Repair/extract damaged teeth.
- Surgically repair fractures.

INFORMATION FOR CLIENTS

- Young animals should never be left alone. Protect animals from accidental electrical burns and ingestion of caustic chemicals by confining them when they cannot be watched.
- Keep pets fenced or on a leash to decrease roaming and the possibility of gunshot wounds.
- Limit cats' access to thread and needles.
- Avoid feeding bones to dogs and cats.
- Seek veterinary assistance for any head injury.

- Advances in dental repair make it possible to cap and repair damaged teeth.
- Animals can do well with loss of large amounts of tongue tissue.

SALIVARY MUCOCELE

The salivary mucocele is the most common clinically recognized disease of the salivary glands in dogs, although it may also occur in cats secondary to trauma. A mucocele is an accumulation of excessive amounts of saliva in the subcutaneous tissue and the consequent tissue reaction that occurs. This disease occurs most often in dogs between the ages of 2 and 4 years; German Shepherds and Miniature Poodles are the most commonly affected. The initial cause of the accumulation is usually unknown. Owners report a history of a slowly enlarging, fluid-filled, nonpainful swelling on the neck. The animal may have respiratory distress or difficulty swallowing secondary to the partial obstruction of the pharynx. In cats, a ranula (a large fluid-filled swelling under the tongue) may be seen.

CLINICAL SIGNS
- Slowly enlarging, nonpainful, fluid-filled swelling on the neck or under the tongue
- Reluctance to eat
- Difficulty swallowing
- Blood-tinged saliva
- Respiratory distress

DIAGNOSIS
- Clinical signs
- Paracentesis shows a stringy, blood-tinged fluid with a low cell count.
- Sialography by retrograde infusion of a water-soluble angiographic contrast material (Renografin: 0.055 to 0.11 ml/kg body weight [BW]) into the duct of the salivary gland

TREATMENT
- Aspiration of the fluid
- Surgical drainage
- Removal of the gland followed by placement of a Penrose drain for 5 to 7 days

INFORMATION FOR CLIENTS

- The cause of the development of mucoceles in animals is unknown, although trauma may be involved in some cases.
- Without removal of the gland excessive amounts of fluid will continue to accumulate.
- Some cases may spontaneously resolve.

ORAL NEOPLASMS

Oral neoplasms are relatively common in the dog and the cat, with malignant melanomas and squamous cell carcinomas being the most common. In general, older patients are more commonly affected, and males are at an increased risk for malignant melanoma and fibrosarcoma. Dogs with heavily pigmented oral mucosa are also at higher risk of malignant melanoma than dogs having pink oral mucosa.

Benign neoplasms such as papillomas and epulides are seen in the dog. Papillomas, pale-colored cauliflower-like growths, are viral in etiology and may be surgically removed or may regress spontaneously. Epulides occur in the gingiva near the incisor teeth. They are generally slow growing but some may be locally invasive and involve bone destruction.

Malignant melanomas are rapidly growing tumors characterized by early bone involvement. They metastasize early to the lungs and regional lymph nodes. These lesions are dome shaped or sessile and may be black, brown, mottled, or unpigmented.

Squamous cell carcinomas are ulcerative, erosive neoplasms. They invade the mucosa and often the bone and metastasize to regional lymph nodes.

Treatment for oral neoplasia includes surgical removal, chemotherapy, and/or radiation therapy. The prognosis for malignant oral neoplasms is guarded to poor.

CLINICAL SIGNS

- Signs depend on location and size of growth
- Abnormal food prehension
- Increased salivation
- Halitosis
- Tooth loss
- Oral pain

DIAGNOSIS
- Diagnosis is by histology of the mass.
- CBC/serum chemistries
- Radiographs to rule out visceral metastases and to evaluate bone involvement
- Lymph node biopsy

TREATMENT
- Surgical excision with a 2 cm tumor-free margin
- If bone is involved or metastasis is suspected, a hemimaxillectomy or a hemimandibulectomy should be performed. Extensive bone and soft tissue removal can be performed without harm to the animal.
- Radiation therapy
- Chemotherapy:
    Cisplatin in dogs for squamous cell carcinomas
    Doxorubicin/cyclophosphamide for cats with squamous cell carcinomas and fibrosarcomas

INFORMATION FOR CLIENTS
- Prognosis for animals with malignant neoplasia is guarded to poor even with aggressive treatment.
- Benign lesions have a good prognosis following surgical resection and/or radiation therapy.
- Animals (especially cats) having maxillectomies or mandibulectomies may need nutritional support such as a feeding tube.

ESOPHAGEAL DISEASE

Diseases of the esophagus include megaesophagus (see Chapter 9), esophagitis/gastroesophageal reflux, vascular ring anomalies (see Chapter 2), and foreign body obstruction.

ESOPHAGITIS/GASTROESOPHAGEAL REFLUX

Esophagitis is an inflammation of the esophageal wall and is most often associated with contact of irritants with the mucosa of the esophagus. Acids, alkalis, drugs, and hot materials can produce lesions of varying severity in the esophagus. The extent of the lesion will depend on (1) the type of material, (2) the length of contact with the mucosal surface, and (3) the integrity of the esophageal mucosal barrier. Physical trauma by foreign bodies or chemical damage from chronic vomiting may predispose the esophagus to further damage.

The esophagus has a great ability to withstand injury. The mucosa-gel barrier, tight cell junctions, and a bicarbonate-rich layer all serve to protect the mucosal lining from damage. One of the most common causes of esophagitis is gastroesophageal reflux (GER). In normal animals, the lower esophageal sphincter prevents reflux of gastric contents back into the esophagus. Gastric acid, pepsin, and trypsin found in gastric fluid will damage the mucosal lining if allowed to remain in contact with it for prolonged periods. Once inflammatory damage to the esophagus has occurred, lower esophageal sphincter function becomes abnormal, perpetuating the problem.

CLINICAL SIGNS
- Anorexia
- Dysphagia
- Excessive salivation
- Regurgitation
- Concurrent signs of respiratory disease (calicivirus in cats)

DIAGNOSIS
- Endoscopy will demonstrate mucosal inflammation and the presence or absence of ulceration. The lower esophageal sphincter may be open abnormally in animals with GER. Fluoroscopy may be required to document actual reflux.

TREATMENT
- The goal of treatment is to decrease inflammation and to protect the lining from further damage.

INGESTION OF IRRITANT SUBSTANCES
- *Do not* induce vomiting. It may cause further damage to the esophagus.
- Administer neutralizing compounds (e.g., activated charcoal, egg white, sodium bicarbonate, olive oil) or check the container for information on accidental ingestions.
- Bathe or flush the skin with water to prevent further ingestion.
- Use intestinal absorbants such as activated charcoal to decrease further toxic effects.

- Rest the esophagus by withholding food and water for several days.
- You may need a gastrostomy tube in severe cases.
- Sucralfate: Dissolve a 1-g tablet in 10 ml of warm water then give 5 to 10 ml orally three times daily.
- Antibiotics: Broad spectrum
- Corticosteroids: Use at antiinflammatory doses.

GASTROESOPHAGEAL REFLUX

- Dietary changes: Recommend weight loss and use of a high-protein, low-fat diet to normalize gastric emptying.
- Sucralfate (see previous section for dose)
- Histamine H_2-receptor blockers or proton pump blockers:
  Cimetidine (Tagamet): 1 to 4 mg/kg t.i.d.
  Ranitidine (Zantac): 2 mg/kg t.i.d.
  Omeprazole (Prilosec): 0.7 mg/kg daily
- Metoclopramide (Reglan): 0.2 to 0.4 mg/kg t.i.d. to q.i.d. to increase lower esophageal pressure and esophageal motility

INFORMATION FOR CLIENTS

- Prevent access to irritant materials such as cleaning liquids, chemicals, paint thinners, and medications. Avoid feeding foods heated in the microwave because they may contain hot spots that can result in burns to the esophagus; always stir well to mix and cool.
- Proper weight management will prevent pets from becoming obese. A good exercise program will help most pets keep their weight in the proper range.
- Healing of the esophagus is a slow process and treatment may be required for a long period of time.

ESOPHAGEAL OBSTRUCTION

Ingestion of nondigestible foreign objects is more common in the dog than in the cat, with young animals being more likely to be affected. Bones and small play toys commonly lodge at the thoracic inlet, cardiac base, or distal esophagus. The degree of damage to the esophagus depends on the size of the object, the shape, and the time spent in contact with the esophageal mucosal lining.

Prompt removal is important to prevent serious damage. Endoscopy will allow the clinician direct visualization of the object and most foreign bodies can be removed by endoscopic retrieval. Those that cannot be removed orally can often be pushed into the stomach and removed surgically. Surgical removal of foreign objects directly from the esophagus has a less favorable prognosis because of the poor healing qualities of the esophagus and the potential for stricture formation.

CLINICAL SIGNS
- Exaggerated swallowing movements
- Increased salivation
- Restlessness
- Retching
- Anorexia
- History of chewing on foreign objects

DIAGNOSIS
ENDOSCOPY
- Use a flexible or rigid endoscope. A basket or retrieval forceps may be used to grasp the object for removal. Once the object is removed the mucosal lining of the esophagus can then be examined for damage.

RADIOLOGY
- If the object is radiopaque, it may be seen on radiographs. Contrast material can be used to outline radiolucent objects. Iodated contrast agents should be selected if a perforation is suspected.

TREATMENT
- Prompt removal of the foreign object is imperative.
- Fast the animal for 24 to 48 hours following removal to allow the esophagus to rest and begin healing.
- After 48 hours, resume feeding with soft foods for several days.
- Treat the esophagitis that may be present (see previous section).
- If damage to the esophagus is extensive, placement of a percutaneous endoscopic gastrostomy (PEG) tube may be required.

INFORMATION FOR CLIENTS
- Limit access to bones and small toys that can be swallowed.
- String and needles present a special hazard for cats.
- The prognosis is usually good for these animals if serious damage to the esophagus can be prevented.

DISEASES OF THE STOMACH

The stomach is located in the left cranial abdomen and stores ingesta, mixing it with gastric juices and then propelling it into the duodenum at a controlled rate. Anatomically, the stomach wall is composed of three layers of tissue: the mucosal (epithelial) lining, the muscular (smooth muscle) layer, and the serosa. The mucosal lining contains glands that secrete mucus, parietal glands that secrete hydrochloric acid, chief cells that secrete pepsinogen, and argentaffin cells that secrete gastrin. Gastric mucosal cells also secrete bicarbonate.

Gastric motility depends on two motor control centers in the stomach plus external control from the autonomic nervous system. Emptying of solids depends on caloric density and pyloric resistance. The presence of fats and proteins will delay gastric emptying.

The normal bacterial flora of the stomach consists of spirilla (*Helicobacter* sp. and *Gastrospirillum hominus*). In addition, cats may have a nonpathogenic *Chlamydia* living in the mucosal lining of their stomachs.

Disruption of the gastric mucosal barrier (the mucosal lining, mucous coating, and bicarbonate layer) or motility disorders can result in damage to the stomach. The most commonly seen disorders include gastritis, both acute and chronic; ulceration; foreign body obstruction; gastric dilatation/volvulus; hypermotility; and neoplasia.

ACUTE GASTRITIS

One common cause of vomiting in dogs and cats is acute gastritis. Causes of acute gastritis include diet (spoiled food, change in diet, food allergy, or food intolerance), infection (bacterial, viral, or parasitic), and toxins (chemicals, plants, drugs, or organ failure). Ingestion of foreign objects may also result in gastritis. Whatever the cause, once the mucosa is damaged, inflammation occurs and clinical symptoms develop.

CLINICAL SIGNS
- Anorexia
- Acute onset of vomiting
- Presence or absence of dehydration
- Presence or absence of painful abdomen
- History of dietary change, toxin ingestion, or infection
- History of internal parasites

DIAGNOSIS
- Based on history and the physical examination
- A complete blood count may indicate a stress leukogram and dehydration.
- Serum chemistries to rule out metabolic imbalances or organ failure

TREATMENT
- Nothing by mouth for 24 to 36 hours.
- Fluid therapy may be given subcutaneously (SQ) or IV, depending on the severity of the dehydration (66 ml/kg/day plus additional fluids to offset loss from vomiting).
- After 36 hours, start feeding with a low-fat diet such as Hill's I/D canned food, low-fat cottage cheese (1 part) and boiled rice (2 parts), or well-drained boiled meat (1 part) and boiled rice (3 parts).
- Antiemetics:
  Chlorpromazine—dog: 0.5 mg/kg intramuscularly (IM) q 8 h; cat: 0.5 mg/kg IM q 8 h
  Metoclopramide: 0.2 to 0.5 mg/kg q 6 h PO, IM, SQ
- Antibiotics are seldom necessary but are frequently prescribed because vomiting can upset the normal flora of the gastrointestinal tract.

INFORMATION FOR CLIENTS
- Avoid abrupt changes in diet for your pet. Mix the new diet with the old and slowly increase the amount of the new food in the diet for the first week. After the first week you may feed only the new food.
- If your pet vomits two to three times, take it off food and water for 24 hours. If the vomiting continues, call your veterinarian.
- Dogs and cats do not need a varied diet. They can be satisfied with the same food every day. Avoid feeding table scraps and human food because these can cause gastritis.
- Avoid giving pets objects that can be swallowed or chewed into small, abrasive pieces.

IMMUNE-MEDIATED INFLAMMATORY BOWEL DISEASE (CHRONIC GASTRITIS, ENTERITIS, COLITIS)

This type of bowel disease is the result of the accumulation of inflammatory cells within the lining of the small intestine, stomach, or the large bowel and is seen most commonly in cats, although it occurs in dogs also. The range of symptoms reported with this disease is related to the location and type of infiltrate. The cause of the inflammatory infiltrates within the lining of the gastrointestinal tract is unknown but is most likely related to chronic antigenic stimulation of some type. Diagnosis is made from intestinal and gastric biopsies. Treatment begins with daily administration of corticosteroids along with metronidazole. If the patient has a good response, as measured by decreased clinical symptoms, then the amount administered may be slowly decreased over 1 to 2 weeks. More severe cases may require azathioprine or cyclophosphamide. Hypoallergenic diets should be prescribed for these animals.

CLINICAL SIGNS
- Chronic vomiting
- Weight loss
- Diarrhea
- Straining to defecate, mucus in stool

DIAGNOSIS
- Complete blood count
- Serum chemistries
- Urinalysis
- Fecal sample for culture if bacterial problem suspected
- Feline leukemia/feline immunodeficiency virus testing
- All of the above are required to rule out other causes of chronic vomiting and diarrhea.
- Endoscopic evaluation of the stomach, small intestine, and colon lining along with biopsies of each area provide a definitive diagnosis and confirm the type of infiltrate present.

TREATMENT
- Prednisone: 1 to 2 mg/kg every 12 hours for several months then in tapering doses for maintenance
- Azathioprine: 2 mg/kg PO daily for 1 week then every 48 hours
- Cyclophosphamide: 50 mg/m^2 (reserved for severe cases)
- Sulfasalazine — Dog: 25 to 50 mg/kg PO q 8 to 12 h; cats: 10 to 20 mg/kg PO q 8 to 12 h. Best for disease involving the colon.
- Hypoallergenic diet: A diet free of preservatives or additives, with a highly digestible protein source not commonly used for the species (rabbit, lamb, tofu, chicken, etc.). Homemade diets that are rice based work well. Commercial diets are now available.

INFORMATION FOR CLIENTS

- The diagnosis of inflammatory bowel disease requires a complete laboratory workup to rule out other causes of the clinical symptoms.
- A definitive diagnosis requires an intestinal biopsy.
- Therapy will be required for the life of the animal.
- The pet will require a special diet for life. The owner must eliminate all other food sources from the animal's diet. This may mean eliminating flavored vitamins, treats, and table food.
- The immunosuppressive drugs used to treat this disease have side effects in animals. Polyuria, polydipsia, polyphagia, weight gain, and skin and urinary infections may occur. The animal must be closely monitored by the veterinarian, and the lowest possible dose of antiinflammatory drug must be used.
- Nursing care for these animals includes keeping the perianal area clean and soothed (if diarrhea is present).

GASTRIC ULCERATION

Gastric ulceration and erosion is commonly the result of drug therapy in the dog and cat. Nonsteroidal antiinflammatory drugs (NSAIDs) are the most commonly implicated drugs, producing ulceration in humans as well as in dogs. These drugs, which include aspirin, ibuprofen, flunixin meglumine, and phenylbutazone, disrupt the normal gastric mucosal barrier resulting in ulceration. Stress, as seen in severely traumatized animals or animals in strenuous training, can also result in gastric erosion.

CLINICAL SIGNS

- Signs vary from asymptomatic to vomiting blood
- Anemia
- Edema
- Melena
- Anorexia
- Abdominal pain
- Septicemia if perforation has occurred

DIAGNOSIS
RADIOLOGY

- Contrast studies using multiple positions and barium sulfate (unless a perforation is suspected) may show ulcerations in the mucosa of the stomach.

ENDOSCOPY

- Allows direct observation of ulcerated areas; more expedient for assessing the extent of the problem

TREATMENT

- Fluid therapy if animal is dehydrated
- Restrict oral intake of food and fluids.
- Oral antacids containing aluminum hydroxide or magnesium hydroxide given 4 to 6 times daily may help.
- H_2 antagonists: Cimetidine, 5 to 10 mg/kg PO b.i.d. to t.i.d.; ranitidine, 2.2 mg/kg PO b.i.d.
- Omeprazole: 0.7 to 2 mg/kg PO s.i.d.
- Sucralfate (Carafate): 0.5 to 1 g PO b.i.d. to q.i.d. Sucralfate binds to the ulcer site, protecting it from damage. It can also bind other drugs and should not be given at the same time as other medications.
- Misoprostol: 1 to 5 µg/kg PO b.i.d. to t.i.d.; this drug protects against gastric mucosal damage and decreases acid secretion.

INFORMATION FOR CLIENTS

- Do not use NSAIDs in animals without veterinary supervision.
- *Never* administer ibuprofen, naproxen, or aspirin to a dog or cat without a prescription.
- If your veterinarian prescribes these medications for your pet, ask if you may give the medication with a meal or antacids to prevent gastric irritation.

GASTRIC DILATION/VOLVULUS (GDV)

GDV is primarily a disease of 2- to 10-year-old large and giant breed, deep-chested dogs, but it can occasionally occur in small breeds. The exact mechanism for the disease remains unclear, but diet and exercise have been implicated in its development. Delayed gastric emptying, pyloric obstruction, aerophagia, and engorgement may predispose dogs to dilation and volvulus. Recent studies indicate that affected dogs may have gastric dysrhythmias that predispose them to GDV.

The stomach is similar to a bag with openings at each end. As the stomach fills with air, food, and/or fluid, the outflow tracts can become occluded. Further distension results in simple dilation (an air-filled stomach), or the air-filled stomach may twist along its longitudinal axis (volvulus). The pylorus usually passes under the stomach and comes to rest above the cardia on the left side of the abdomen. The enlarged tympanic stomach pushes against the diaphragm, making breathing difficult and blocking venous return of blood through the hepatic portal vein and the posterior vena cava. The increased luminal pressure within the gastric wall results in ischemia and subsequent necrosis of the wall.

The spleen may also be involved and can become congested. Endotoxins that accumulate in the gastrointestinal tract activate the inflammatory mediators. The end result is the development of hypovolemic, endotoxic shock in patients with GDV.

CLINICAL SIGNS
- Weakness, collapse
- Depression
- Nausea
- Nonproductive retching
- Hypersalivation
- Abdominal pain and distension (distension may not be evident in very large dogs)
- Increased heart rate and respiratory rates

DIAGNOSIS
- History and physical examination reveal a depressed, weak animal with prolonged CRT and abnormal mucous membranes.
- Radiographs of right lateral view best define torsion. The stomach will appear air filled (Fig. 3-3). The pylorus will be gas filled and seen dorsal and cranial to the gastric fundus. A compartmentalization is frequently observed between the pylorus and the fundus.
- Electrocardiographic monitoring may indicate a ventricular arrhythmia or sinus tachycardia.
- Complete blood counts and serum chemistries are necessary for correction of electrolyte/pH imbalances and for proper fluid therapy.

TREATMENT
- The goal of treatment is to decompress the stomach, stabilize the patient, and prepare the patient for surgical intervention.

AGGRESSIVE TREATMENT OF SHOCK
- 14- to 16-gauge jugular catheter or two cephalic catheters should be placed.

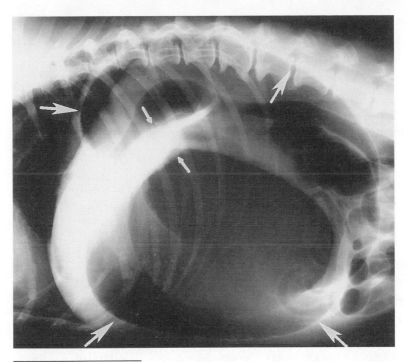

FIGURE 3-3.   Lateral radiograph of a dog with gastric dilation/volvulus. Stomach is dilated *(large arrows)* and there is a "shelf" of tissue *(small arrows),* demonstrating that the stomach is malpositioned. Radiographs obtained from the right lateral position seem superior to those of other views in demonstrating this shelf. If the stomach were similarly distended but not malpositioned, the diagnosis would be gastric dilation. (From Nelson RW, Couto CG: *Small animal internal medicine,* ed 2, St Louis, 1998, Mosby.)

- Crystalloid IV fluids at 45.5 mg/kg over a 15-minute period
- Corticosteroids: 10 mg/kg IV (Solu-Delta, Cortef) or flunixin meglumine (0.5 to 1 mg/kg IV)
- Bicarbonate: Total CO_2 is <12 mEq. The dose may be calculated using the formula: body weight (kg) × (12 − patient's HCO_3^-) × 0.3. Give this amount IV over 30 to 60 minutes.

ALLEVIATE DISTENTION

- In an emergency situation, an 18-gauge needle may be used as a trocar to relieve the pressure in the stomach. Clip and scrub a small area caudal to the costal arch. Insert the needle through the skin and into the stomach to allow gas to escape.

- Pass a stomach tube and decompress the stomach. Care must be taken not to perforate the already compromised stomach or the distal esophagus. Place the animal in sternal or lateral recumbency and use a large-bore tube.
- If surgery must be delayed, placement of a temporary gastrostomy tube can be performed.
- Perform gastric lavage to remove all the remaining food and fluid.

Antibiotics
- Antibiotics targeted against gram-negative/anaerobic microorganisms are given IV (cefoxitin 20 mg/kg IV q 6 h; or ampicillin 20 mg/kg IV q 6 h).

Continuous monitoring of the ECG
- Treat ventricular arrhythmias with lidocaine (2 mg/kg IV) if necessary. If the arrhythmia is lidocaine responsive, a constant rate infusion of 30 to 80 µg/kg per minute can be established. If the arrhythmia is not lidocaine responsive, procainamide can be given IV at a dose of 6 to 10 mg/kg in 2-mg/kg boluses every 5 minutes. If effective, continue constant rate infusion (CRI) at 25 to 40 µg/kg per minute.

Potassium
- Potassium supplementation may be required if potassium levels are less than 3 mEq/L.

Surgical correction
- Surgery should be considered as soon as the patient is stable.

Postoperative nursing care
- Continuous ECG monitoring for at least 24 hours.
- Serial observation of hemodynamic parameters; mean arterial pressure (MAP) >70 mm Hg, systolic pressure >110 mm Hg
- Pain management: Oxymorphone 0.05 to 2 mg/kg q 4 h or to effect
- Monitor urine output/fluid input using a closed catheter system.
- Monitor serum electrolytes and acid-base status every 8 hours.
- Continue antibiotics.
- Gastric atony and ileus may produce vomiting: Metoclopramide 2 to 5 mg/kg q 8 h SQ to control.

- Maintain good body temperature and turn patient frequently to prevent skin and muscle damage.
- Provide parenteral nutritional support if vomiting. Start oral fluids in small volumes at 12 hours postoperatively if not vomiting. Offer low-fat canned food the day after surgery unless resection of the stomach or bowel has been performed.

INFORMATION FOR CLIENTS
- Avoid feeding large dogs one huge meal per day. Several small meals will prevent gastric overload.
- Limit exercise immediately after eating.
- Feed a high-quality protein, low-fat diet. Avoid easily fermentable diets.
- The average hospital stay for dogs with GDV is about 3 to 7 days.
- The mortality rate for this disease is between 15% and 18%.
- Surgical correction and tack-down procedures (gastropexy) are *not* a guarantee against future episodes of GDV.

GASTRIC NEOPLASIA

The most common malignant canine gastric neoplasm is the adenocarcinoma. This type of tumor is most commonly found in older animals, and because the clinical signs are relatively nonspecific (vomiting and weight loss), the tumor may be well advanced before it is diagnosed.

Gastric lymphoma is the most commonly diagnosed feline gastric tumor. Polyps and gastric leiomyomas, both benign tumors, may also be seen in dogs and cats.

CLINICAL SIGNS
- Weight loss
- Vomiting with or without blood
- Obstruction
- Usually seen in older animals

DIAGNOSIS
- Endoscopy to locate the lesion. A biopsy is required for diagnosis. In some cases, a full-thickness biopsy from a surgical approach may be required for a definitive diagnosis.

TREATMENT
- Surgical removal is the treatment of choice; however, many tumors are too advanced at the time of diagnosis and are inoperable. Cats with a single lesion (e.g., lymphosarcoma) usually respond well to removal of the single mass.
- Chemotherapy: Long-term response is not good.
- Radiation is not successful for treatment of these tumors.

INFORMATION FOR CLIENTS
- The prognosis for malignant gastric tumors is guarded to poor. This is a fatal disease.
- Supportive care, control of vomiting, and maintenance of a good nutritional status is important for keeping these animals comfortable.

DISEASES OF THE SMALL INTESTINE

Disease of the small intestine involves impairment of the absorptive villous surface of the small intestine, which results in diarrhea, malabsorption, and weight loss. Types of intestinal damage may include villous atrophy, disruption of the microvilli, and disruption or defects in villous proteins. Diarrhea, defined as an increase in frequency, fluidity, and volume of defecation, may result anytime the flux of fluid or nutrients across the absorptive membrane is altered. It may be classified in several ways: acute or chronic; *osmotic* (resulting from decreased digestion or absorption that increases the osmotic solute load in the bowel), *secretory* (due to hypersecretion of ions), *exudative* (resulting from an increased permeability with loss of plasma proteins), or *dysmotility* (resulting from abnormal motility).

Diarrhea may also be classified with respect to the causative agent: parasitic, viral, bacterial, or dietary intolerance/sensitivity.

ACUTE DIARRHEA

Acute diarrhea is one of the most commonly seen types of diarrhea in the small animal clinic. Frequently, the cause is a change of diet, drug therapy, or any stressful situation that may result in disruption of the normal bacterial flora within the bowel. Acute diarrhea is easily managed with supportive and symptomatic treatment.

CLINICAL SIGNS
- Abrupt onset of diarrhea
- Presence or absence of vomiting
- Otherwise, a normal-appearing animal

DIAGNOSIS
- Rule out other causes of diarrhea
- Fecal sample for direct and flotation examination
- HCT to monitor hydration

TREATMENT
SUPPORTIVE
- Replace fluid and electrolytes (SQ, PO, or IV)
- Nothing by mouth for 24 to 48 hours. Water is allowed if the animal is not vomiting.
- Intestinal absorbants: Pepto-Bismol 1 ml/5 kg q 8 h
- Loperamide: 0.1 mg/kg q 6 h
- Antibiotics: Choose a broad-spectrum drug.

DIETARY
- Start on a bland, low-fat diet after 24 to 48 hours.
- I/D (Hill's) canned food
- Chicken/rice or beef/rice: Boil the meat and drain well. Mix 1 part meat with 4 parts boiled rice. Feed small amounts for 2 to 3 days until stool returns to normal then return to regular diet.

PARASITIC DIARRHEA

Intestinal parasites may be the primary cause of diarrhea in the small animal patient. The technician should review the life cycles and pathophysiology of the common intestinal parasites. Common parasite eggs and protozoans are shown in Fig. 3-4.

CLINICAL SIGNS
- Diarrhea
- Presence or absence of blood
- Presence or absence of vomiting
- Weight loss

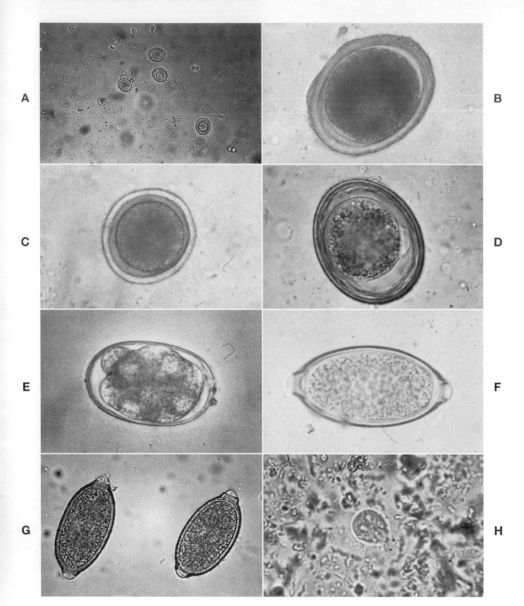

FIGURE 3-4.   Common parasite eggs and oocysts found in dog and cat feces. **A,** Unsporulated oocysts of *Isospora* species. *I. canis* (large oocysts) and *I. bigemina* (small oocysts) are present. **B,** Egg of *Toxocara canis.* **C,** Characteristic egg of *Toxocara cati* is similar in structure to that of *T. canis* but smaller in diameter. **D,** Eggs of *Toxascaris leonina.* These eggs have a smooth outer shell and hyaline, or "ground glass," central portion. **E,** These eggs of hookworm species may represent one of several genera that parasitize dogs and cats: *A. caninum, A. tubaeforme, A. braziliense,* and *U. stenocephala.* **F,** Characteristic egg of *Truchuris vulpis.* **G,** Egg of *Eucoleus aerophilus (Capillaria aerophila).* **H,** Cysts of *Giardia* species.

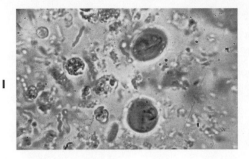

FIGURE 3-4, CONT'D.   I, Motile tropho-
zoite of *Giardia* species. (From Hendrix
CM: *Diagnostic veterinary parasitology,*
ed 2, St Louis, 1998, Mosby.)

- Poor hair coat
- Listlessness
- Anorexia

DIAGNOSIS
- Fecal sample for direct and flotation examination

TREATMENT
ANTHELMINTICS FOR A SPECIFIC PARASITE
- Fenbendazole: 50 mg/kg orally for 3 consecutive days
- Pyrantel pamoate: 5 mg/kg orally, repeat in 10 to 14 days

ANTIPROTOZOAL MEDICATION
- Giardia: Metronidazole, 25 to 30 mg/kg b.i.d. for 5 to 10 days orally; albendazole, 25 mg/kg b.i.d. for 2 days
- Coccidia: Albon, 55 mg/kg oral loading dose followed by 27.5 mg/kg for 9 days

VIRAL DIARRHEA

Viral diarrheas are seen in young animals and in animals not vaccinated against the common offenders such as parvovirus, distemper, coronavirus, or feline panleukopenia virus.

CLINICAL SIGNS
- Diarrhea with or without blood
- Presence or absence of vomiting
- Patient may or may not be febrile
- Anorexia
- Depression

DIAGNOSIS

- Parvovirus: ELISA test (CITE or IDEXX)
- Canine distemper titer
- Panleukopenia with a white blood cell count <500 WBC/μl

TREATMENT

SUPPORTIVE

- Intravenous fluids
- Antidiarrheal therapy
- Antibiotics having gram-negative spectrum

PREVENTION

- Vaccination

NURSING CARE

TECH ALERT

These animals are immunosuppressed.
- Avoid giving fluids SQ because infections and skin necrosis can develop.
- Keep the animal clean and dry. Avoid letting fecal matter collect on the coat or the perianal skin.
- Keep the animal warm. If using a heating pad, take care to turn the animal frequently to prevent thermal injury to the skin.
- Wear protective clothing and shoe covers when handling these animals. These animals and all materials that they come in contact with may be infectious to other clinic patients.
- Have an isolation area in the clinic especially for these patients. Keep all necessary materials for treatment and maintenance of these patients in the isolation area. Never bring the patient into the main clinic area. All disposable materials from the contaminated area should be disposed of directly into the outdoor trash receptacle.

INFORMATION FOR CLIENTS

- The sick animal may infect other dogs or cats in the household.
- Coronavirus diarrhea is usually not fatal.
- The prognosis with parvovirus depends on the severity of the disease (estimated by the decrease in the WBC count).

- The mortality for canine distemper is about 50%, and the prognosis for feline panleukopenia (feline distemper) is guarded to poor.
- These viruses can be spread by contact with feces. Avoid areas where high concentrations of unvaccinated animals may congregate (parks, boarding kennels, beaches, dog shows). Make sure that your pet is properly vaccinated, and make sure that your kennel, animal hospital, dog show, and so on, require current vaccination records on all animals.

BACTERIAL DIARRHEA

Pathogenic bacteria produce intestinal disease by invading and damaging the intestinal epithelium by releasing enterotoxins that stimulate secretions, attaching to the mucosal surface, and/or producing cytotoxins. Bacteria such as *Salmonella, Shigella, Campylobacter,* and some strains of *Escherichia coli* invade the mucosa, whereas *Clostridium* produces cytotoxins. *Staphylococcus* induces hypersecretion and also invades the mucosal lining.

CLINICAL SIGNS
- Diarrhea with or without blood
- Patient may or may not have fever
- Anorexia

DIAGNOSIS
- Rule out parasites with a fecal examination.
- The presence of gram-negative, slender, curved rods in stained fecal smears or S-shaped motile organisms with darting or spiral movement in fresh saline smears can indicate *Campylobacter.*
- Fecal cytotoxin assay for *Clostridium* with a titer >1:20
- *E. coli*: No reliable way to serotype this organism in animals is available.

TREATMENT
- Oral antibiotics (if disease is severe)
    Enrofloxacin: 5 mg/kg b.i.d.
    Trimethoprim/sulfa: 15 mg/kg b.i.d.
    Erythromycin: 10 mg/kg t.i.d.
    Metronidazole: 25 to 30 mg/kg b.i.d.
- Fluid and electrolyte replacement (IV or SQ)

> ⚠ **TECH ALERT**
>
> When handling animals, proper hygiene is required to prevent transmission of disease from the animal to the nursing staff and owners.
>
> Hospitalized and stressed animals are at risk of developing *Salmonella* infections. Asymptomatic carriers may break out with clinical disease when stressed.
>
> Animals kept in close confinement in shelters, pounds, and kennels may develop *Campylobacter* infections, which can be transferred to humans.

DIETARY INTOLERANCE/SENSITIVITY DIARRHEA

Dietary-induced intestinal disease is common in small animals. The etiology may be immune mediated (dietary sensitivity) or nonimmunologic (dietary intolerance). Identification of a specific cause is often difficult. Dietary sensitivity can be diagnosed after a complete clinical and dietary history and a thorough laboratory examination is performed to rule out other causes of vomiting, diarrhea, abdominal discomfort, and weight loss. Endoscopic biopsies should be used to assess the damage to the intestinal mucosa.

Dietary intolerance is seen in animals that are unable to handle certain substances in their diet such as carbohydrates, fats, or milk products. This condition is most often seen in animals who are fed large amounts of table food or who raid the garbage for scraps. Some animals are intolerant of processed animal foods containing milk products or large amounts of fats.

Symptoms of dietary indiscretion are also seen in pets that ingest foreign materials such as paper, tin foil, rubber bands, and other household substances.

CLINICAL SIGNS
- Diarrhea
- Vomiting
- Abdominal pain or discomfort
- Weight loss

DIAGNOSIS
- History of sensitivity to specific foods
- History of a recent diet change
- Physical examination and lab work to rule out all other causes of symptoms

Complete blood count (CBC) and serum chemistries
Fecal examination
Radiographs to rule out partial bowel obstructions
Fecal culture and sensitivity
Trypsinlike immunoreactivity test

TREATMENT

- Dietary trial: Feeding of an exclusion diet for a minimum of 6 weeks. This diet should contain a protein source not usually eaten by the animal (e.g., chicken, rabbit); the diet should contain no milk products and no preservatives (Table 3-1).
- Oral prednisone 0.5 to 1 mg/kg b.i.d. for 2 to 4 weeks followed by a dose reduction at 2-week intervals.

INFORMATION FOR CLIENTS

- Prevent pets from gaining access to garbage and other foreign objects that can result in irritation to the bowel.
- Commercial diets containing novel protein sources are readily available. These must be fed for adequate periods of time to see clinical response (2 to 3 months).
- Treats and some medications contain additives to which the pet may be sensitive. Avoid using these items while your pet is on a restricted protein source diet.
- Longhaired pets should have the hair shaved around the rectum to prevent loose stool from accumulating.
- It may take lots of trial and error to determine the cause of this problem. Be patient with your veterinarian.

CHRONIC ENTEROPATHIES

Chronic, inflammatory bowel disease in the dog and cat is commonly seen in small animal practice. Lymphocytic-plasmocytic enteritis, seen in both the dog and the cat, represents the most common form of this disease. Chronic antigenic stimulation within the intestinal lumen (from a variety of causes) results in excessive infiltration of the lamina propria with lymphocytes and plasma cells. Infiltration results in damage to the mucosa and abnormal intestinal absorption. Management and treatment are aimed at eliminating the antigen and decreasing the immune response.

TABLE 3.1. Home-prepared diets for intestinal disease* (approximately 10-kg dog)

HIGHLY DIGESTIBLE LOW-FAT EXCLUSION DIETS (SINGLE-SOURCE PROTEIN)

SUPPLIES 675-700 KCAL 20%-34% OF CALORIES FROM PROTEIN, 46%-48% FROM CHO, AND 19%-22% FROM FAT

Lamb	*Venison*	*Rabbit*
6 oz lean lamb	6 oz venison	6 oz rabbit
No corn oil	2 teaspoons corn oil	1 teaspoon corn oil
10 oz boiled white rice	10 oz boiled white rice	10 oz boiled white rice
1 teaspoon dicalcium phosphate	1 teaspoon dicalcium phosphate	1 teaspoon dicalcium phosphate
1 teaspoon lite salt	1 teaspoon lite salt	1 teaspoon lite salt
½ capsule "Centrum" adult multivitamins	½ capsule "Centrum" adult multivitamins	½ capsule "Centrum" adult multivitamins

HIGHLY DIGESTIBLE MODERATE- AND HIGH-FAT DIETS

SUPPLIES 680 KCAL

(33% OF CALORIES FROM PROTEIN, 37% OF CALORIES FROM CHO, AND 30% FROM FAT [CHICKEN])

(33% OF CALORIES FROM PROTEIN, 24% FROM CHO, AND 43% FROM FAT [BEEF])

Chicken (moderate-fat)	*Beef* (high-fat)
6 oz chicken	6 oz hamburger (lean)
8 oz boiled white rice	6 oz boiled white rice
2 teaspoons corn oil	No corn oil
1 teaspoon dicalcium phosphate	1 teaspoon dicalcium phosphate
1 teaspoon lite salt	1 teaspoon lite salt
½ capsule "Centrum" adult multivitamins	½ capsule "Centrum" adult multivitamins

*Ingredients for each diet should be well mixed and cooked in a microwave oven or casserole before serving.

CLINICAL SIGNS

- Usually these are nonspecific
- Chronic, intermittent vomiting with or without diarrhea
- Listlessness
- Weight loss
- Older animals
- Polyuria or polydipsia
- Borborygmus
- Halitosis
- Flatus
- Symptoms are progressive, becoming more frequent over time.

---

❶ TECH ALERT

Vomiting hairballs is an important clinical sign of disease in cats.

DIAGNOSIS

PHYSICAL EXAM

- Usually unremarkable
- Edema or ascites may be seen if serum protein levels are low.

LABORATORY TESTS

- Complete blood count/serum profile: Panhypoproteinemia, neutrophilia, hypocalcemia (cats may have normal serum protein)
- Fecal examination to rule out intestinal parasites
- Biopsy to identify lymphocytic-plasmacytic infiltrates within the lamina propria (customarily reported as mild, moderate, or severe)

TREATMENT

MEDICAL

- Oral prednisolone: 0.5 to 1.0 mg/kg q 12 h for a month followed by 50% reduction every 2 weeks.
- Azathioprine: 1 mg/kg daily in dogs and 0.3 mg/kg daily in cats for 3 to 9 months. Monitor WBC counts every 2 to 4 weeks while on medication.
- Metronidazole: 10 to 20 mg/kg b.i.d. for 2 to 4 weeks, then once daily.
- Intestinal protectants: Sucralfate 0.25 to 0.5 g t.i.d.; cimetidine

5 mg/kg t.i.d. to decrease erosive disease and protect against excessive protein loss in dogs.

- Vitamin therapy to replace fat-soluble vitamins A, D, K, and B

DIETARY

- Limit carbohydrates, avoid lactose. (Rice is a good source of carbohydrates, especially for dogs.)
- Restrict dietary fats.
- Feed a good quality protein (animal derived).
- Dietary therapy alone is seldom successful in the cat, although there are commercial hypoallergenic diets available that may be tried.

INFORMATION FOR CLIENTS

- Treatment for this disease may be prolonged and expensive.
- A cure is not usually obtained.
- Pets on antiinflammatory therapy will need to be monitored on a routine basis (white blood cell counts) to prevent the occurrence of bone marrow suppression.

INTESTINAL LYMPHANGIECTASIA

This chronic protein-losing intestinal disease of dogs is characterized by impaired intestinal lymphatic drainage resulting from obstruction of normal lymphatic flow. The backup of lymph releases fluid into the intestinal lumen resulting in a loss of lipids, plasma protein, and lymphocytes.

CLINICAL SIGNS

- Edema and effusion
- Ascites/hydrothorax
- Presence or absence of light-colored diarrhea
- Weight loss, progressive emaciation
- Progressive symptoms

DIAGNOSIS

- CBC and serum chemistry profile showing lymphopenia, hypocholesterolemia, hypoglobulinemia, decreased serum albumin and globulin levels, and hypocalcemia
- Biopsy showing chyle-filled lacteals and intestinal lymphatics with ballooning distortion of villi and mucosal edema

TREATMENT
- The aim of treatment is to decrease the loss of intestinal protein.

MEDICAL
- Prednisolone: 1 to 2 mg/kg b.i.d.; adjust after remission is achieved.
- Metronidazole: 10 to 20 mg/kg b.i.d.

DIETARY
- Choose a food with minimal fat and good quality protein source.
- Divide food into 2 or 3 feedings.
- Supplement diet with fat-soluble vitamins.

SURGERY
- Surgery may be necessary to relieve any obvious obstructions to lymph flow.

INFORMATION FOR CLIENTS
- This disease is usually progressive and, although remissions can be achieved, most dogs will relapse and finally succumb to protein depletion, diarrhea, or severe effusions.
- Treatment may be prolonged and will require dietary management to achieve remission.
- There is no cure for most animals.

INTESTINAL NEOPLASIA

Intestinal adenocarcinomas account for about 25% of all intestinal neoplasms in the dog and 52% in the cat. Lymphosarcomas, the next most common neoplasm, account for 10% of the gastrointestinal neoplasms in the dog and 21% in the cat. Mast cell tumors occur in the cat as well. Clinical signs are usually progressive and are related to the location and growth rate of the tumor. Widespread metastasis may occur. Adenocarcinomas typically occur in the older animal, whereas lymphosarcomas may be found in animals of any age, although middle-age to older animals are most commonly affected.

CLINICAL SIGNS
- Weight loss
- Signs of partial gastrointestinal obstruction
- Presence or absence of melena

- Signs of malabsorption, maldigestion with or without vomiting and diarrhea
- Abdominal discomfort
- Anorexia

DIAGNOSIS
PHYSICAL EXAM
- Abdominal mass may be palpable in the intestines or the intestinal wall may feel thickened. Mesenteric lymph nodes may be enlarged.

RADIOGRAPHY
- Contrast studies may show mucosal irregularity, thickened wall, abnormal luminal diameter ("apple core" sign).

BIOPSY
- Endoscopic biopsy is possible for lesions in the upper GI, but surgical biopsy is usually required for most animals.

LABORATORY TESTS: CBC/SERUM PROFILE
- Anemia
- Hypoproteinemia
- Leukocytosis with a left shift
- Serum tests may show the involvement of other organ systems.

TREATMENT
- Surgical removal of the tumor if possible
- Dogs respond poorly to chemotherapy; cats may do well on COP (cytoxan, oncovin, prednisolone) protocol.
- Supportive care should include good nutritional management and transfusions if needed.
- Antibiotics to control bacterial overgrowth during chemotherapy
- For mast cell tumors: Prednisone, cimetidine, antibiotics

INFORMATION FOR CLIENTS
- The prognosis for adenocarcinoma is poor with mean survival times (with treatment) of 7 months to 2 years.
- Cats with lymphosarcoma respond well to chemotherapy with remissions lasting up to 2 years.

- For animals with cancer, supportive care is important. Nutritional support is critical. High quality, easily digestible diets are required to maintain cellular repair.

DISEASES OF THE LARGE BOWEL

The large bowel may be divided into the cecum, the colon, and the rectum. The cecum is a small, sigmoid-shaped diverticulum found near the ileocolic junction. The colon can be divided into the short, ascending portion (the right side of the abdomen); the transverse portion (cranial abdomen); and the long, descending portion (the left side of the abdomen). Histologically, the wall is similar to that of the small intestine with no villi. Crypts of Lieberkühn contain epithelial, mucous, and endocrine cells. Large numbers of goblet cells in the colon produce mucus when stimulated.

The main function of the colon in the dog and the cat is water and electrolyte reabsorption. The colon also serves to store feces while microorganisms ferment undigested material and produce vitamins K and B.

The most common signs of large bowel disease are diarrhea, straining to defecate, and blood in the stool. Diagnosis is by colonoscopy and histopathologic evaluation of mucosal samples.

Inflammatory Bowel Disease

A diagnosis of inflammatory bowel disease (IBD) is often made when an excessive number of inflammatory cells are found in mucosal samples of the gastrointestinal system of the dog and cat. The etiology is unknown but is probably multifactorial. Colonic inflammation disrupts mucosal integrity and results in decreased absorption of sodium and water. Inflammation also increases motility, resulting in more frequent defecation.

CLINICAL SIGNS
- Diarrhea with little weight loss
- Increased frequency of defecation and decreased fecal volume
- Tenesmus
- Hematochezia
- Increased mucus
- Mild fever

DIAGNOSIS

LABORATORY TESTS

- CBC/serum chemistry profile to rule out other causes of diarrhea. Usually no consistent pattern of abnormalities are seen with IBD.
- Complete fecal exam to rule out parasites

RADIOGRAPHS

- May show gas-filled loops of intestine

HISTOPATHOLOGY

- Increased numbers of lymphocytes and plasma cells in the lamina propria of the large bowel

TREATMENT

MEDICAL

- Sulfasalazine:
    - *Dogs*: 20 to 50 mg/kg to maximum of 1 g q 8 h. Decrease dose after fourth week of no diarrhea. Decrease the dose 50% after 4 additional weeks free of diarrhea. Side effects: Vomiting—give with food. Keratoconjunctivitis sicca (KCS) may develop over a period of 6 to 8 months of treatment.
    - *Cats*: Use with caution owing to sensitivity to salicylates: 10 to 20 mg/kg q 12 h
- Prednisone: 1.0 to 2.0 mg/kg q 24 h (dogs); 0.5 to 2.0 mg/kg q 24 h (cats)
- Mesalamine: 11 to 22 mg/kg q 8 h (dogs); 11 mg/kg q 8 h (cats) (may also cause KCS)
- Metronidazole: 10 to 20 mg/kg q 8 h
- For case refractory to treatment: Azathioprine 2 mg/kg q 24 h (dogs); 0.3 mg/kg q 48 h (cats)
- Tylosin: 5 to 100 mg/kg q 12 h

DIETARY

- Hypoallergenic diets low in fat are recommended.
- Hill's Science Diet–Maximum Stress
- Prescription diet (dermatology diet [d/d], canine diet [c/d], reducing diet [r/d])
- Home diets low in fat and high in fiber

INFORMATION FOR CLIENTS
- Treatment for this condition may be prolonged.
- The goal of treatment is control of symptoms.
- Animals suffering from this disease may have to be taken outside many times daily to defecate.

INTUSSUSCEPTION

The cause of intussusception is usually idiopathic, but can be the result of parasite infection, foreign bodies, infections, and neoplasia. Intussusception occurs when the smaller, proximal segment of the intestine at the ileocolic junction invaginates into the larger, more distal segment of the large bowel. This "telescoping" produces a partial to complete blockage and compromises the blood supply to the segments causing bowel necrosis.

CLINICAL SIGNS
- Vomiting
- Anorexia
- Depression
- Diarrhea with or without blood in dogs

DIAGNOSIS
- Palpation of a sausagelike mass in the cranial abdomen
- Ultrasound shows multilayered concentric rings representing bowel wall layers.

TREATMENT
- Surgical reduction or resection of necrotic bowel
- Restore fluid and electrolyte balance if necessary.
- Broad-spectrum antibiotics postsurgically
- Restrict solid food for 24 hours after surgery, then resume a bland diet for 10 to 24 days to allow healing of the intestinal wall.

INFORMATION FOR CLIENTS
- Recurrence of intussusception is infrequent.
- The prognosis depends on the amount of bowel involved and the extent of damage to that bowel.
- Puppies should be treated for parasites on a proper schedule to prevent

bowel irritation and intussusception. Ask your veterinarian for preventive treatment recommendations.

MEGACOLON

Although the literature reports megacolon to be an uncommon condition, it is seen frequently in our practice. The typical patient is a middle-age to older, obese cat that is presented for straining to defecate. Some cats are able to pass a liquid stool containing blood and/or mucus. These cats are usually dehydrated and may be vomiting. Palpation reveals a markedly distended colon packed with firm feces. Radiographs confirm the diagnosis. Medical and dietary management are usually unrewarding in the long term, and surgery should be considered in cases with repeat episodes. The etiology of this disorder has been thought to involve a defect in the neurostimulation mechanism that promotes colon evacuation. Other causes, such as hypokalemia, hypothyroidism, pelvic deformities, or prolonged, severe colonic distension for any reason, can disrupt normal motility and result in megacolon. Sixty-two percent of cases are idiopathic.

CLINICAL SIGNS
- Straining to defecate (must be distinguished from straining to urinate in the male cat)
- Vomiting
- Weakness
- Dehydration
- Anorexia
- Small, hard feces or liquid feces with or without blood, mucus

DIAGNOSIS
- Physical examination: Distended colon is filled with firm, packed feces.
- Radiographs show colon width greater than the length of the lumbar vertebra.
- CBC/serum chemistries show dehydration, increased HCT; may also show dysfunction of other organ systems.

TREATMENT
MEDICAL
- Stool softeners may be effective only if constipation is mild.
  Dulcolax: 1 to 2 pediatric suppositories or 5 mg q 24 h PO

Colace: 1 to 2 pediatric suppositories or 50 mg q 24 h PO
- Lactulose (Cephulac): 0.5 ml/kg q 8 to 12 h
- Enemas: 5 to 10 ml/kg warm water mixed with 5 to 10 ml/cat of dioctyl sodium succinate and gentle digital removal of feces if necessary
- Propulsid (Cisapride): 0.1 to 0.5 mg/kg q 8 to 12 h PO or 0.15 to 1 mg/kg q 8 to 12 h PO if moderately constipated

❗ TECH ALERT

Propulsid has recently been removed from the market owing to serious medical complications in humans. Cats do well on the medication and experience few side effects.
- Correct dehydration and electrolyte imbalances.
- Provide antibiotics to protect against sepsis through the damaged colonic wall.
- Treat any underlying disease.

DIETARY
- Increase fiber in the diet.
- Add raw, canned pumpkin to diet.
- Use high fiber diet (prescription r/d or w/d).
- Provide soft food (canned).
- Increase water intake by salting food.

SURGERY
- Subtotal colectomy if disease is refractory to medical management.

HOSPITAL CARE
- Anesthesia is required for severely constipated cats. These cats should be rehydrated and have electrolyte imbalances corrected before anesthesia to avoid problems.
- Manual removal of the feces from the colon must be performed with care. Use a well-lubricated, gloved finger, and take care not to scrape or use excessive pressure against the already compromised colon wall.
- Radiograph the cat after feces removal to ensure the colon is empty.
- Postevacuation: Use a soothing ointment or cream around the rectum, and make sure the patient is wiped clean and dried. Keep the patient warm.
- Patients will pass excess enema fluid after the procedure. Make sure the perineal area is kept clean while in the hospital.

INFORMATION FOR THE CLIENT

- Without surgery, this problem will be a recurring problem in most cats.
- Medical treatment will be for the life of the cat.
- After surgical correction, cats do well and often pass fairly normal feces within several months.

CONSTIPATION (CANINE)

Many times owners will call the veterinarian asking what they can give their constipated animals. Because true constipation is uncommon in dogs and cats, the technician (and the veterinarian) should be wary of prescribing laxatives without examining the patient.

The presence of foreign objects, tumors, pelvic injury, anal sac abscesses, urinary obstruction, dehydration, and a number of other factors can result in the failure to pass feces. Giving laxatives in the presence of mechanical obstruction or metabolic dysfunction may only complicate the situation. The owner should be advised to have the animal examined before medicating.

CLINICAL SIGNS

- Straining to defecate
- Anorexia
- Passing small amounts of very hard, dry stool
- Presence or absence of vomiting

DIAGNOSIS

- Palpation of a distended colon with an otherwise normal physical examination
- Radiographs confirm that the colon is full of feces with no physical obstruction.
- Serum chemistries and CBCs should be done to rule out other organ disease and to monitor hydration.
- Rectal palpation assures adequate pelvic canal opening.

TREATMENT

- Enema with warm water and dioctyl sodium succinate (DSS)
- Oral laxatives: Dulcolax, Colace
- Restore fluid and electrolyte balance as necessary.
- Manual removal of feces under anesthesia if required

INFORMATION FOR CLIENTS

- Prevent access to small foreign objects that may obstruct the bowel if swallowed (bones, small toys, rocks, etc.).
- Make sure pets always have access to water.
- Do not treat "constipated" animals without a complete physical examination by your veterinarian.
- High fiber diets may help pets prone to constipation.

LIVER DISEASE

The liver plays a major role in a number of biologic processes within the animal body. It has been estimated that the liver carries out at least 1500 functions essential for survival. Because the liver has a large functional reserve and good regenerative capabilities, liver injury must be severe before laboratory tests reveal the presence of disease.

Signs of liver disease are usually vague in the early stages. These signs include anorexia, vomiting, diarrhea or constipation, weight loss, polyuria, polydipsia, and pyrexia. Cats often display hypersalivation. Some animals may develop bleeding tendencies due to vitamin K malabsorption. (Vitamin K requires bile acids for absorption.) Jaundice may develop as the disease progresses.

Liver diseases can be categorized as follows: drug- or toxin-induced liver disease, infectious liver disease, feline hepatic lipidosis, neoplastic liver disease, and congenital portosystemic shunts.

DRUG- OR TOXIN-INDUCED LIVER DISEASE (ACUTE)

Acute liver failure occurs when at least 70% to 80% of functional liver mass is injured. The liver is most susceptible to damage from ingested toxins because the liver receives 100% of the portal venous blood from the stomach and the intestine. Toxins may be specific for hepatocytes or may simply be toxic to all cells, but reach the hepatocytes first. Some are made more toxic after they are metabolized inside the hepatocytes.

The species and sex of the animal, dose of toxin, route of administration, and duration of exposure are all factors affecting the extent of liver damage. Although toxicosis is not a frequent occurrence in dogs and cats, drugs that are most commonly implicated are acetaminophen, phenobarbital, caparsolate, antifungals, diethylcarbamazine, anabolic steroids, and halothane or Metofane. Acute onset of hepatic disease usually results from an overdose of these medications, whereas chronic damage may occur with long-term use at clinical doses.

CLINICAL SIGNS
- Acute onset of symptoms
- Anorexia
- Vomiting
- Diarrhea/constipation
- Polyuria (Pu)/Polydipsia (Pd)
- Presence or absence of jaundice
- Melena and/or hematuria
- Signs of central nervous system (CNS) involvement: Depression, ataxia, dementia, blindness, seizures, and coma

DIAGNOSIS
- History of recent drug administration
- Palpation of painful liver, which may be increased in size
- Serum chemistries:
    - Markedly increased alanine aminotransferase (ALT)
    - Increased alkaline phosphatase (ALP)
    - Increased total bilirubin
    - Increased fasting and postprandial serum bile acids
    - Hypoglycemia
    - Hyperammonemia
    - Coagulopathy
- Radiographs
- Ultrasound shows decreased echogenicity of the liver that is usually diffuse.
- Liver biopsy: Unless coagulopathy is suspected

TREATMENT
ANTIDOTES
- Available only for acetaminophen
- Induce vomiting
- Give activated charcoal
- N-acetylcysteine 20% IV

SUPPORTIVE THERAPY
- Aggressive replacement of fluids and electrolytes (IV) with B complex vitamins added (1 ml/L)

- Glucose may be added if needed (2.5% to 5%).
- Vitamin K therapy
- Cimetidine 5 mg/kg SQ, IV or ranitidine 2 mg/kg SQ, IV
- Antibiotics: Amikacin 10 mg/kg q 8 h and ampicillin 22 mg/kg q 8 h *or* enrofloxacin 2.5 mg/kg IM q 12 h and ampicillin

NUTRITIONAL SUPPORT
- Dogs: Hill's Prescription Canine k/d or u/d
- Cats: Hill's Prescription Feline k/d

DRUG- OR TOXIN-INDUCED LIVER DISEASE (CHRONIC)

Long-term use of drugs such as anticonvulsants (phenytoin, phenobarbital, primidone), glucocorticoids, diethylcarbamazine, methimazole, antifungals, and NSAID-like drugs such as carprofen and phenylbutazone can result in chronic liver damage.

CLINICAL SIGNS
- Weight loss
- Anorexia
- Weakness
- Ascites
- Jaundice
- Pu/Pd

DIAGNOSIS
- History of long-term use of a hepatotoxic drug
- Serum chemistries:
    Increased ALP (2 to 12 times normal)
    Increased ALT (2 to 5 times normal)
    ALT increase >ALP increase
    Increased serum bile acids
    Hypoalbuminemia
    Hypocholesterolemia
- Liver biopsy: Hepatocellular hypertrophy, cirrhosis (anticonvulsants), and vacuolated hepatocytes (steroids) may suggest hepatotoxic disease.

TREATMENT
- *Stop* medication!
- Begin a low-protein diet.

- Force-feeding or gastric feeding tube may be required if animal is not eating.
- Maintain adequate hydration.
- If neurologic signs are present: Lactulose, dogs 2.5 to 15 ml PO q 8 h; cats 2.5 to 5 ml PO q 8 h
- Antibiotics as in acute hepatotoxicity

NURSING CARE

- If using an indwelling feeding tube, make sure to flush with clear water after each feeding. If the tube becomes clogged, a small amount of carbonated beverage can be placed into the tube for flushing out the obstruction. Keep the tube and point of entry through the skin clean. Dogs and cats require 50 to 100 ml of water daily. Animals must receive adequate calories known as the *resting energy requirement (RER)*. This may be calculated using the formula:

$$RER = (30 \times BW_{kg}) + 70$$

where *BW* is the animal's body weight in kilograms.
- Animals that are ill or under stress will require more energy than normal, healthy animals. Therefore, you must multiply the calculated RER by a factor of 1.2 to 1.5 (the value depends on the amount of stress to the animal) to compensate for this increased energy requirement. The equation then becomes:

$$1.5 \times (RER)$$

or

$$1.5 \times ([30 \times BW_{kg}] + 70)$$

- Hill's Prescription Diet a/d or Eukanuba Veterinary Diet Recovery Formula (canned) can be used to prepare a gruel or for liquid feeding.

INFECTIOUS CANINE HEPATITIS

Infectious canine hepatitis (ICH) is caused by canine adenovirus 1 (CAV-1) and has long been recognized as a cause of hepatic necrosis in dogs. Owing to effective vaccination programs, the disease is uncommon today. However, unvaccinated dogs and feral animals are still susceptible to the virus. Infection occurs via the oronasal route. Viral replication occurs in the tonsils and regional lymph nodes. Viruses released into the body localize in the liver.

CLINICAL SIGNS

- Petechial hemorrhages
- Lethargy
- Fever >103° F
- Depression
- Pale mucous membranes
- Abdominal pain
- Anorexia
- Corneal opacities ("blue eye")
- Bloody diarrhea
- Hepatomegaly

DIAGNOSIS

- CBC: Neutropenia, lymphopenia with WBC <2500 in severe cases; thrombocytopenia
- Serum chemistry: Increased ALT
- Serum titers for ICH: Elevated and increasing

TREATMENT

- IV fluids
- Force feeding if necessary
- Blood transfusion if necessary

INFORMATION FOR CLIENTS

- Vaccination is the best prevention for this disease. Make sure your pet is vaccinated properly.
- This is a viral infection, and it will not respond to antibiotic therapy. Supportive therapy is the only means of treatment that will help the animal.

LEPTOSPIROSIS

Leptospirosis is caused by infection with antigenically distinct serovars of *Leptospira interrogans*. Domestic and wild animals serve as reservoirs of infection for humans and other animals. Recently, cases of leptospirosis have been on the increase. Serotypes previously not associated with clinical disease are now being isolated from infected dogs. Serovars *canicola* and *icterohemorrhagica* have classically been the cause of canine renal and liver disease. At present, serovars *pomona, grippotyphosa,* and *bratislavia* are also being isolated from dogs with symptoms of leptospirosis. Typically dogs are incidental hosts for these sero-vars with skunks, raccoons, opossums, and pigs being the natural hosts.

Clinical symptoms of leptospirosis include acute renal failure with or without hepatic involvement. Leptospirosis should be considered in any dog showing these symptoms.

Animals with leptospirosis may pose a health hazard for humans and other animals. Infected animals should be isolated, and anyone handling them should wear protective clothing and practice good hygiene. Laboratory technicians should take care when handling body fluids.

CLINICAL SIGNS
- Acute renal failure
- Dehydration
- Vomiting
- Fever
- Increased thirst
- Reluctance to move
- Jaundice
- Peracute shock and death

DIAGNOSIS
SEROLOGY
- Microscopic agglutination test: A fourfold rise in titer over 4 weeks is a positive diagnosis.
- Fluorescent antibody test will not identify serovar.
- Polymerase chain reaction allows identification of serovar but is not readily available.

COMPLETE BLOOD COUNT
- Leukocytosis, thrombocytopenia

SERUM CHEMISTRY
- Increased blood urea nitrogen (BUN), creatinine
- Increased ALT
- Bilirubinuria

TREATMENT
SUPPORTIVE TREATMENT
- IV fluids
- Furosemide if oliguric

ANTIBIOTICS
- Penicillin: 25,000 to 40,000 U/kg q 24 h IV or IM for 14 days followed by doxycycline
- Doxycycline: 5 to 10 mg/kg PO b.i.d. for 14 days to eliminate the carrier state

INFORMATION FOR CLIENTS
- Animals with leptospirosis are contagious to humans and other animals.
- Supportive care is important.
- Treatment and diagnosis are expensive.
- Vaccinations do not protect your dog from other serovars that it may come in contact with.

CHOLANGIOHEPATITIS

Cholangiohepatitis is a common hepatobiliary disorder of cats, but it is less common in dogs. This condition is a complex of disorders involving cholangitis, cholangiohepatitis, and biliary cirrhosis.

Bile duct inflammation leads to hepatocyte involvement, which progresses to cirrhosis. The exact cause is unknown, although ascending biliary infections from the gastrointestinal tract and immune-mediated mechanisms have been suggested. Persian cats seem to have a predisposition for this disorder. A chronic pancreatitis is commonly seen in cats with cholangiohepatitis.

CLINICAL SIGNS
- Anorexia
- Depression
- Weight loss
- Vomiting
- Dehydration
- Fever
- Jaundice
- Ascites as the disease progresses
- Hepatomegaly

DIAGNOSIS
COMPLETE BLOOD COUNT
- Neutrophilia with a left shift
- Mild, regenerative anemia

SERUM CHEMISTRY
- Mild to moderate increase in ALT
- Normal to increased ALP
- Mild to moderate increase in δ-glutamyltransferase (GGT)
- Normal to increased fasting serum bile acids
- Hypoalbuminemia in later stages
- Decreased BUN in later stages

RADIOLOGY
- Hepatomegaly, choleliths may be observed.

LIVER BIOPSY
- Cellular infiltrates in and around bile ducts with or without portal fibrosis is the definitive diagnosis.

TREATMENT
- Antibiotics based on culture/sensitivity
  Ampicillin: 22 mg/kg PO, IV, SQ q 8 h for as long as 3 months
  Amoxicillin: 20 mg/kg PO, SQ bid
  Metronidazole: 25 to 30 mg/kg PO q 12 h
- Ursodeoxycholic acid: 10 to 15 mg/kg PO q 24 h
- Prednisolone: 2.2 to 6.6 mg/kg PO q 24 h for 1 to 2 weeks then taper to 2 to 4 mg/kg q 48 h
- Fluid and electrolyte corrections
- Nutritional support as for other liver disorders
- Vitamin therapy

INFORMATION FOR CLIENTS
- The prognosis for this disease is variable.
- Treatment may be prolonged and expensive.
- There may be permanent damage to the liver.

FELINE HEPATIC LIPIDOSIS (IDIOPATHIC)

Idiopathic hepatic lipidosis (IHL) is the most common hepatopathy seen in cats. IHL affects adult, obese cats of any age, sex, or breed. The exact cause of the disease is unknown, but stress seems to trigger the syndrome. Any diet change, boarding, illness, or environmental change resulting in anorexia can precipitate the event. If the anorexia is prolonged for longer than 2 weeks, an imbalance between the breakdown of peripheral lipids and lipid clearance within the liver can occur, resulting in excess accumulation of fat within hepatocytes. Other proposed mechanisms for this disease include hormonal abnormalities (leptin, insulin), impaired formation and release of very-low-density lipoprotein (VLDL) from the liver, and decreased oxidation of fatty acids in the liver. The resulting clinical signs are those of hepatic failure. Early diagnosis and aggressive treatment is important for recovery. Complete recovery has been achieved in about 60% to 65% of reported cases.

CLINICAL SIGNS
- Anorexia
- Obesity
- Weight loss (often >25% of body weight)
- Depression
- Sporadic vomiting
- Icterus
- Mild hepatomegaly
- Presence or absence of bleeding tendencies (i.e., tendency to hemorrhage spontaneously from gums, petechial hemorrhages on ears, abdomen)

DIAGNOSIS
COMPLETE BLOOD COUNT
- Nonregenerative anemia
- Stress neutrophilia
- Lymphopenia

SERUM CHEMISTRY
- Markedly increased ALP
- Increased ALT, aspartate aminotransferase (AST)
- Hyperbilirubinemia
- Hypoalbuminemia
- Increased serum bile acids

RADIOGRAPHS
- Liver mildly enlarged

ULTRASOUND
- Liver hyperechoic when compared with the falciform fat

LIVER BIOPSY

- Severely vacuolized hepatocytes. Fat is confirmed using Oil red O stain on formalin-fixed liver tissue (Fig. 3-5).

TREATMENT

NUTRITIVE SUPPORT

- High-protein, calorie-dense diet
- Usually requires a feeding tube (Fig. 3-6)
    Nasogastric tube for short-term, liquid diets
    Gastrostomy tubes are best if cat can handle anesthesia.
    Gastroesophageal tube is not well tolerated by cats.
- Tubes may need to remain in place for up to 3 to 6 weeks (no less than 10 days).
- Diets for nutritional support include Hill's Prescription a/d, c/d, p/d, Purina CNM Feline CV Formula, Iams Nutritional Recovery Formula.
- Mix 1 oz of water with 1 oz of food.
- Daily caloric needs may be calculated using the formula:

$$RER = 1.5 ([30 \times BW_{kg}] + 70)$$

Example: a 5-kg cat would require 330 Kcal/day or about ⅘ of a 15.5-oz can of c/d.

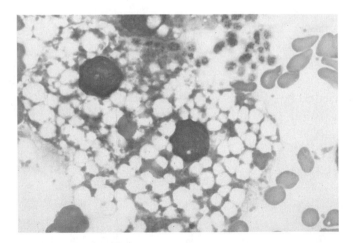

FIGURE 3-5. Feline fatty liver. Swollen hepatocytes contain small clear vacuoles representing lipid accumulation and fine intracytoplasmic granular clumps of bile pigment. (From Baker R, Lumsden JH: *Color atlas of cytology of the dog and cat,* St Louis, 2000, Mosby.)

- Divide the total amount into six feedings for the first several days to allow the stomach to adjust to the presence of food. Then slowly decrease the number of feedings to three per day.
- Flush tube with water before and after feeding (10 to 15 ml).
- If vomiting occurs, feed a smaller volume, warm the food, or provide medication.

MEDICATIONS

- IV fluids to maintain hydration
- Potassium supplement (if necessary)

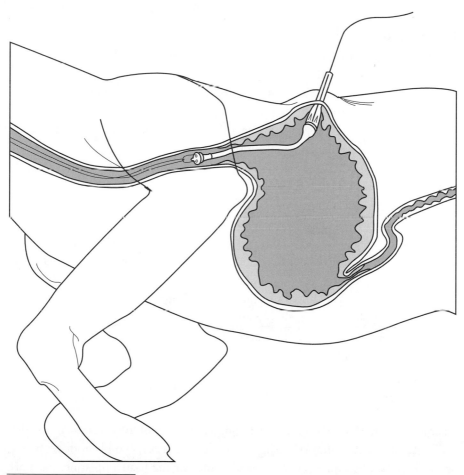

FIGURE 3-6. Gastrostomy tube.

- Metoclopramide SQ about 15 minutes before feeding at a dose of 0.4 mg/kg
- Diazepam as an appetite stimulant is seldom successful long term.

MONITORING

- Recheck weekly to assess progress.
- CBC, serum chemistries every 2 weeks. Expect to see decreases in ALP, ALT in 1 to 2 weeks.
- Owners may have to skip a tube feeding as laboratory values become normal. Many cats enjoy the tube feedings and will not eat on their own unless challenged. Try special treats or favorite foods. When the cat is eating well, the tube may be removed.
- Withhold food for 8 hours before tube removal and 12 hours after removal.

NURSING CARE

- Feeding tubes must be flushed before and after feeding.
- Keep tube capped.
- Keep site clean, and apply antiseptic ointment around the tube to protect the skin.
- After removing the tube, instruct the client on how to clean and care for the wound until healing is complete.

INFORMATION FOR CLIENTS

- Avoid stress in obese cats.
- Early intervention is essential.
- A cat that usually eats well then stops eating is at risk. This means owners should monitor the food intake under stressful conditions and have the cat seen immediately if problems arise.
- Cats do not do well with frequent diet changes.
- Prevent obesity by feeding your cat properly.
- Although the prognosis is guarded, with early intervention and aggressive treatment, the cure rate is around 60% to 65%.

NEOPLASIA

Primary and metastatic tumors are a significant cause of liver disease in the dog and cat. Metastatic tumors arising from the pancreas, lymph nodes, spleen, mammary glands, bone, lungs, thyroid gland, or the gastrointestinal tract are more common than primary liver tumors. Primary tumors are usually epithelial in nature and are derived from hepatocytes or biliary epithelium. Hepatocellular adenomas and adenocarcinomas are most common in dogs, whereas bile duct neoplasms are most common in cats.

Carcinomas may occur in three forms: massive—a single large mass in one liver lobe; nodular—discrete nodules in several liver lobes; and diffuse—infiltration throughout a large mass of liver tissue. Metastases are frequent.

Primary hepatic neoplasm is most common in animals over 10 years of age. Clinical signs are usually nonspecific and vague and may not be noticed until the tumor is advanced. Surgical removal of a single mass is the treatment of choice. Nodular and diffuse neoplasms respond poorly to chemotherapy and carry a poor prognosis.

CLINICAL SIGNS

- Anorexia (especially in cats)
- Lethargy (especially in cats)
- Weight loss
- Pu/Pd
- Vomiting (especially in dogs)
- Abdominal distension (dogs)
- Jaundice
- Presence or absence of diarrhea
- Presence or absence of bleeding
- Pale mucous membranes
- Hepatomegaly

DIAGNOSIS

COMPLETE BLOOD COUNT

- Anemia, usually nonregenerative

SERUM CHEMISTRY

- Increased ALT, ALP (mild to marked) (cats may have a normal ALP)
- Hyperbilirubinemia
- Hypoalbuminemia
- Hypoglycemia
- Increased serum bile acids
- Hyperglobulinemia
- Azotemia (especially in cats)

RADIOLOGY
- Symmetric or asymmetric hepatomegaly
- Presence or absence of ascites
- Rule out metastasis to thorax with a chest radiograph.

ULTRASOUND
- Focal, multifocal, or diffuse changes in echogenicity of the liver

BIOPSY
- Best done through laparotomy or fine needle aspiration for diffuse lesions

ABDOMINAL TAP
- May show tumor cells

TREATMENT
SURGICAL
- Remove affected lobe if a single lesion is present.

CHEMOTHERAPY
- Primary liver tumors respond poorly to chemotherapy. Better response may be obtained with metastatic tumors.

SUPPORTIVE
- Correct fluid and electrolyte imbalances.
- Maintain a good nutritional level.
- Treat symptoms of nausea and diarrhea.

INFORMATION FOR CLIENTS
- These tumors carry a guarded to poor prognosis.
- Survival times of 195 to 1025 days have been reported for single masses removed by partial hepatectomy.
- Chemotherapy is unsuccessful for treatment of these cancers.
- Early detection affords the best chance for survival. Routine physical exams are important for your pet.

PORTOSYSTEMIC SHUNTS (CONGENITAL)

Vascular communications between the portal and systemic venous systems that allow blood to bypass the liver are known as portosystemic shunts (PSS).

Because blood carrying toxins from the gastrointestinal tract of animals with this defect bypasses hepatic detoxification, systemic toxin levels increase, resulting in hepatic encephalopathy. The livers of affected animals appear small and atrophied. The PSS may be intrahepatic or extrahepatic, singular or multiple. The single intrahepatic PSS is most common in large-breed dogs whereas the single extrahepatic PSS is most common in cats and small-breed dogs. Intrahepatic PSS is usually caused by failure of the ductus venosus to close at birth. Congenital PSS occurs more commonly in purebred dogs, especially Miniature Schnauzers and Yorkshire Terriers, and in mixed breed cats. Clinical signs usually develop by 6 months of age. Diagnosis is by demonstration of a shunting of portal blood directly into the systemic circulation. Complete or partial ligation of the shunt is the preferred treatment.

CLINICAL SIGNS
Signs of CNS involvement
- Anorexia
- Depression
- Lethargy
- Episodic weakness
- Ataxia
- Head-pressing
- Circling, pacing, blindness
- Seizures
- Coma
- Hypersalivation (cats)
- Bizarre aggressive behavior (cats)

❶ TECH ALERT
Signs may be worse after a high-protein meal.

Gastrointestinal
- Vomiting
- Diarrhea
- Stunted growth and failure to thrive
- Pu/Pd (dogs)

Urinary
- Urate urolithiasis in non-Dalmatians
- Hematuria

- Ammonium biurate crystals in sediment
- Isosthenuria or hyposthenuria if Pu/Pd

DIAGNOSIS
COMPLETE BLOOD COUNT
- Microcytosis
- Target cells
- Poikilocytosis (especially in cats)
- Mild, nonregenerative anemia

SERUM CHEMISTRY
- Hypoproteinemia
- Hypoalbuminemia
- Hypoglycemia
- Decreased BUN
- Increased ALT, ALP (mild, 2 to 3 times normal)
- Increased serum bile acids
- Hyperammonemia

RADIOGRAPHS
- Microhepatia: Can use contrast portography to detect the shunt. Rectal portal scintography is also being used.

TREATMENT
MEDICAL MANAGEMENT
- Seldom successful
- Low-protein diet
- Lactulose
- Neomycin or metronidazole
- Fluid therapy

SURGERY
- Surgical ligation is the preferred treatment. However, total ligation of most shunts may result in serous portal hypertension. In many cases, partial ligation (60% to 80%) can be performed. Closure of the shunt forces blood back through the atrophic liver, resulting in hypertension, abdominal pain, ascites, ileus, endotoxic shock, and cardiovascular collapse. Therefore, partial occlusion is often followed with a second surgery to totally close the shunt, allowing the liver time to adjust to the increased blood flow.

- Animals should be closely monitored for 24 hours postsurgery. If signs of portal hypertension develop, a second surgery should be performed to remove the ligation, and emergency treatment with shock doses of fluids and glucocorticoids along with antibiotics should be given.

POSTSURGICAL MANAGEMENT
- Systemic antibiotics
- Fluid therapy
- Oral lactulose: 15 to 30 ml PO q 6 h (dogs); 0.25 to 1 ml PO (cats)
- Protein-restricted diet

INFORMATION FOR CLIENTS
- The prognosis for resolution of symptoms after surgical ligation of the shunt is excellent.
- Surgery yields the most successful prognosis if performed before the dog is >1 year old.
- The shunt may recanalize after surgery, resulting in relapses (more common in cats).
- Animals with partial ligations of the shunt may require a low-protein diet to avoid clinical signs of hepatic encephalopathy.
- This surgical procedure may be expensive and require a referral center with specialized techniques.

PANCREATIC DYSFUNCTION (EXOCRINE)

The major function of the exocrine pancreas is the secretion of digestive enzymes into the small intestine. It also secretes bicarbonate to neutralize stomach acid, assists in inhibiting bacterial overgrowth in the lumen of the small intestine, and aids in the absorption of vitamin B_{12} and other nutrients.

The pancreas is closely associated with the stomach, liver, and the duodenum. The right lobe lies along the descending duodenum; the left lobe accompanies the pyloric portion of the stomach. The left and right lobes join the body at the cranial end of the duodenum near the liver. Pancreatic ducts open into the duodenum at the major duodenal papilla along with the bile duct and at the minor duodenal papilla.

Digestive enzymes, produced and stored within the acinar cells of the pancreas, are released into the small intestine on a routine basis. When stimulated by the presence of food, the volume of secretion increases. The enzymes are secreted in an inactive form to protect the pancreas from autodigestion. (The inactive forms of the enzymes usually have a prefix of *pro-* or an *-ogen* suffix.) Once in the lumen of the small intestine, the enzymes are chemically activated by enteropeptidase, which removes the protective segment of their polypeptide chain.

The digestive enzymes produced in the pancreas include trypsinogen, chymotrypsinogen, proelastase, procarboxypeptidase, prophospholipase, alpha-amylase, lipase, procolipase, and pancreatic secretory trypsin inhibitor. Amylase and lipase leak from the gland into the blood of normal animals where they are cleared by the kidneys. Clinically, these enzymes are used as a measure of pancreatic health.

PANCREATITIS

Inflammation of the pancreas is known as pancreatitis. It may be acute or chronic and is believed to develop when digestive enzymes are activated *within* the gland, resulting in pancreatic autodigestion. Once autodigestion develops, the gland becomes inflamed, resulting in tissue damage, multisystemic involvement, and, often, death.

Pancreatitis is more prevalent in obese animals. Diets high in fat may predispose animals to the disease. In cats, pancreatitis has been associated with hepatic lipidosis. Drugs such as furosemide, azathioprine, sulfonamides, and tetracycline have been suspected of causing pancreatitis. In addition, edema of the duodenal wall, parasites, tumors, and trauma may also result in pancreatitis.

The disease is unpredictable, with varying levels of severity. Some dogs recover fully whereas others develop fulminating disease and die.

CLINICAL SIGNS
- An older, obese dog or cat with a history of a recent fatty meal
- Depression
- Anorexia
- Vomiting
- Presence or absence of diarrhea
- Dehydration
- Fever
- Presence or absence of abdominal pain
- Shock and collapse may develop

DIAGNOSIS
COMPLETE BLOOD COUNT
- Leukocytosis
- Increased PCV

SERUM CHEMISTRIES
- Azotemia
- Increased ALT
- Mild hypocalcemia
- Hyperlipemia
- Normal to increased amylase, increased lipase
- Increased serum trypsinlike immunoreactivity (TLI), a pancreas-specific test

TREATMENT
- Maintain adequate fluid and electrolyte balance.
- Replace potassium if necessary.
- Suspend all oral intake for 3 to 4 days.
- Antibiotic therapy:
    Trimethoprim-sulfadiazine: 26.4 mg/kg SQ s.i.d. (dogs) and 30 mg/kg SQ q 12 to 24 h (cats)
    Enrofloxacin: 2.5 mg/kg IM q 12 h
- Butorphanol tartrate for analgesia: 0.2 to 0.4 mg/kg SQ q 6 h
- Plasma or albumin: 50 to 250 ml
- 1 to 2 days after vomiting stops, start back on a high-carbohydrate diet. As the animal improves, add a low-fat dietary food.

---

❶ TECH ALERT

Pancreatitis is commonly a postholiday disease. Feeding table scraps from turkey, ham, or roast drastically increases an animal's dietary fat, resulting in acute signs of the disease. Warn your clients to avoid providing these treats!

INFORMATION FOR CLIENTS
- To prevent obesity, avoid overfeeding your pets.
- Feed only low-fat treats.
- Most patients will recover with prompt treatment; however, some dogs may die even with prompt and proper treatment.

EXOCRINE PANCREATIC INSUFFICIENCY (EPI)

Exocrine pancreatic insufficiency develops with a progressive loss of acinar cells followed by inadequate production of digestive enzymes. Because the pancreas has considerable reserves, clinical signs may not develop until 85% to 90% of the secretory ability has been lost. Pancreatic acinar atrophy (PAA) is the most common cause of the disease in dogs. PAA may occur spontaneously in the dog, especially in young German Shepherds, a breed with a genetic predisposition to PAA. In cats, EPI is primarily the result of chronic pancreatitis.

Lack of normal pancreatic secretions affects the mucosal lining of the small intestine and decreases its absorptive power. Bacterial overgrowth that occurs also interferes with absorption. Disruption of the normal acinar architecture of the pancreas may affect insulin production, leading to glucose intolerance.

Clinical signs of EPI include weight loss with a good appetite, diarrhea with a grey, fatty, foul-smelling stool, flatulence, and poor hair coat. Treatment is aimed at replacing digestive enzymes.

CLINICAL SIGNS
- Mild to marked weight loss
- Polyphagia
- Coprophagia and/or pica
- Diarrhea, fatty stool (light in color)
- Flatulence

DIAGNOSIS
COMPLETE BLOOD COUNT
- Normal

SERUM CHEMISTRIES
- Increased ALT (mild to moderate)
- Decreased total lipid
- Serum trypsinlike immunoreactivity; detects both trypsin and trypsinogen; levels are decreased below 2 μg/L in EPI

FECAL TESTS
- Unreliable

FECAL PROTEOLYTIC ACTIVITY
- Decreased in EPI

TREATMENT

- Supplement pancreatic enzymes with each meal—commercial product such as Pancrezyme or Viokase-V (2 tsp/20 kg BW added to food) *or* chopped raw ox or pig pancreas (3 to 4 oz/20 kg BW).
- Low-fiber diet with high digestibility
- Medium chain triglyceride (MCT) oil: 0.5 to 4 tsp/day with food
- Vitamins
    Tocopherol: 400 to 500 IU given once daily with food for 30 days
    Cobalamin: 250 µg IM or SQ every 7 days for several weeks
- Antibiotic therapy to decrease bacterial overgrowth in the small intestine
    Oxytetracycline: 10 to 20 mg/kg q 12 h for 7 to 28 days
    Metronidazole: 10 to 20 mg/kg q 12 to 24 h for 7 days *or*
    Tylosin: 10 mg/kg with each meal
- Prednisolone (1 to 2 mg/kg q 12 h for 7 to 14 days) may be used if response to the above treatments is poor.

INFORMATION FOR CLIENTS

- EPI is irreversible and will require lifelong treatment.
- Pancreatic enzyme replacements are expensive.
- With enzyme replacement, most dogs will regain their weight and the diarrhea will resolve.
- Enzyme replacements must be given with every meal.

RECTOANAL DISEASE

Three conditions involving the recto-anal area are commonly seen in small animal medicine: perineal hernia, perianal gland adenoma, and perianal fistula. Anal sac problems are covered in Chapter 11.

PERINEAL HERNIAS

Perineal hernias, seen most commonly in intact male dogs older than 8 years of age, are associated with neurogenic atrophy of the levator ani muscle and herniation of the rectum and other pelvic organs into the ischiorectal fossa.

CLINICAL SIGNS

- Reducible perineal swelling
- Tenesmus

- Dyschezia (painful or difficult defecation)
- Constipation or obstipation
- Some dogs have signs of urethral obstruction if the bladder is involved.

❶ TECH ALERT
Brachiocephalic breeds show a predisposition to this problem.

DIAGNOSIS
- Rectal palpation will reveal the hernia sac.

TREATMENT
MEDICAL
- Stool softeners such as Colace (DSS) (seldom effective for long-term maintenance)
- Enemas (seldom effective for long-term maintenance)

SURGICAL
- Herniorrhaphy to correct the weakness in the pelvic diaphragm.
- Castration is usually recommended.

INFORMATION FOR CLIENTS
- Keeping the stool well formed but soft may help decrease straining.
- Castration is usually recommended because the role of the hormone testosterone in this disease is unknown.

PERIANAL FISTULAS (ANAL FURUNCULOSIS)

Perianal fistulas are characterized by single or multiple ulcerated sinuses that may involve up to all of the perianal tissue. Their presence can result in pain, bleeding, self-mutilation, dyschezia, and anal stenosis.

CLINICAL SIGNS
- Tenesmus
- Dyschezia, pain on exam
- Fecal incontinence
- Licking of perianal area

- Bleeding
- Foul odor to anal area
- Typically a large-breed dog

DIAGNOSIS
- Examination to rule out anal sac disease and perirectal tumors

TREATMENT
- Medical management is usually not successful.
- Surgical—no one technique has been consistently successful.

INFORMATION FOR CLIENTS
- These animals will have pain around the anal area; be careful to avoid getting bitten when treating them.
- Keep the involved area clean and dry. Spray antibiotics can be used to decrease the level of infection.
- Long-term oral antibiotics may be required for maintenance.

PERIANAL GLAND ADENOMAS

Because growth and development of these tumors are related to plasma androgen levels, 85% are seen in older, intact male dogs. Most lesions are firm, single, or multiple masses that may ulcerate. The lesions may result in intense pruritus and can interfere with defecation. They are not invasive or metastatic.

CLINICAL SIGNS
- Pruritus in anal area
- Bleeding
- Firm nodule in perianal integument, tail root, or the prepuce

DIAGNOSIS
- Palpation and location of lesion
- Biopsy

TREATMENT
- Surgical removal
- Radiation
- Cryosurgery

- Castration results in regression of tumors and decreases the risk of new tumor development.

INFORMATION FOR CLIENTS

- Pets with perianal fistulas or ulcerated adenomas need to be kept clean. Gently cleanse the area daily using a baby wipe or damp cloth.
- Castration of male dogs at an early age can help prevent this disease.

Diseases of the Endocrine System

four

The cells of the body must maintain *homeostasis* (equilibrium) with their internal environment because the chemical processes carried out at the cellular level can only occur under specific conditions. The endocrine system works along with the nervous system to achieve a stable internal environment; each system may work independently or they may act together to accomplish this task. The hypothalamus and the pituitary gland regulate the release of chemical messengers called *hormones* (chemicals secreted directly into the bloodstream) to signal target cells to perform certain functions in response to changes in homeostasis. As hormone concentrations in the blood rise, the system is signaled to reduce hormone production; this *negative feedback system* works much the same way as a thermostat controls the heating system in your home.

Ideally, the glands regulating the release and balance of hormones work continuously to maintain homeostasis. When one or more of these glands work ineffectively, incorrectly, or not at all, the potential for problems develops. The endocrine glands most commonly involved in diseases of small animals are the thyroid gland, adrenal gland, pancreas, parathyroid gland, and gonads (testes and ovaries) (Fig. 4-1).

Diseases affecting the pituitary gland or the hypothalamus result in multiple irregularities in the body; they are only discussed here in the context of their relationship to other syndromes.

THE THYROID GLAND

The thyroid gland is located in the ventral cervical region along the lateral margins of the trachea. The gland is not usually palpable in a normal animal. The gland is composed of follicles that produce the thyroid hormones *triiodo-*

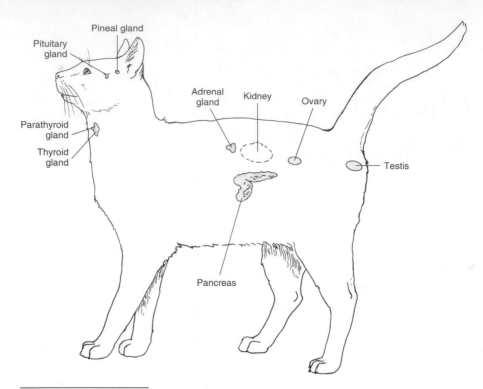

Figure 4-1. Locations of major endocrine glands in the cat. (From McBride DF: *Learning veterinary terminology,* ed 2, St Louis, 2002, Mosby.)

thyronine (T_3) and *tetraiodothyronine* (T_4). These hormones are produced by the follicular cells and stored in the gland until they are needed by the body. A third hormone, *calcitonin,* is produced by the parafollicular cells in the thyroid gland. Calcitonin acts to increase calcium deposition within bone to decrease blood calcium concentration, whereas T_3 and T_4 function to control all of the body's metabolic processes.

Two common diseases of small animals involve the thyroid gland (Fig. 4-2): *hypothyroidism* (insufficient thyroid hormone) and *hyperthyroidism* (excessive thyroid hormone). Hypothyroidism is most commonly seen in the canine (1 in 156 to 1 in 500 animals). Hyperthyroidism is seen primarily in the cat.

Hypothyroid Disease

Primary acquired hypothyroidism is the most common type seen in the dog and usually follows thyroid atrophy or lymphocytic thyroiditis. Central acquired

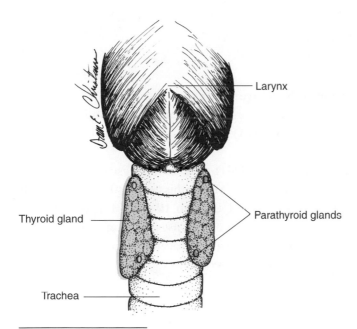

Figure 4-2.   Canine thyroid and parathyroid glands. (From Christenson DE: *Veterinary medical terminology,* Philadelphia, 1997, WB Saunders.)

hypothyroidism is rare and develops when the pituitary or hypothalamus is diseased.

CLINICAL SIGNS

- Breeds predisposed to this disease: Golden Retrievers, Dobermans, Irish Setters, Schnauzers, Cocker Spaniels, and Dachshunds
- Common in middle-age dogs (4 to 10 years of age); female to male ratio is 2.5 : 1
- Weight gain with no change in diet
- Bilaterally symmetrical alopecia; "rat tail" (loss of hair on the tail)

❗ TECH ALERT

Hypothyroid disease and Cushing's disease are the only known diseases that produce this alopecia pattern.

- Dry hair or excessive shedding
- Lethargy

- Anestrus (infertility, testicular atrophy)
- Hyperpigmentation of the skin
- Cold intolerance
- Anemia
- Hypercholesterolemia

DIAGNOSIS

- 66% to 75% of animals will have elevated cholesterol.
- 25% to 40% of animals have a mild, nonregenerative anemia.
- Perform radioimmunoassay (RIA) for T_3 and T_4; normal T_4 concentration is 1 to 4 µg/dl.
- Thyroid stimulating hormone (TSH) tests are expensive and often not available. Recommended doses of TSH for this test are 0.396 U/kg body weight IV or 0.099 U/kg IM or 1 U IV to 10 U IV, IM, or SQ. Take blood sample at 6 hours. The normal response shows an elevation of T_4 concentration greater than 2 µg/dl above baseline concentration.
- Measure thyroid hormone antibody concentration.

TREATMENT

- Life-long supplementation with thyroid replacement hormone
- *Dogs:* Initially use trade-name products at a dose of 0.1 mg/4.5 kg b.i.d. Reevaluate in 4 to 8 weeks for clinical response, and adjust the dose as needed. Some dogs may need only one dose daily.
- *Cats:* 0.05 to 0.1 mg daily. Reevaluate in 4 to 6 weeks and adjust the dose.

PRODUCTS

- Levothyroxine sodium tablets: 0.1 mg, 0.2 mg, 0.3 mg, 0.4 mg, 0.5 mg, 0.6 mg, 0.7 mg, 0.8 mg sizes
- Animal-approved products: Soloxine (Daniels), Thyro-Tabs (Vet-A-Mix), Thyro-Form (Vet-A-Mix) chewable tabs
- Human-approved products: Synthroid (Knoll), 0.025 to 0.3 mg; Levo-T (Lederle), Levothroid (Forest)

INFORMATION FOR CLIENTS

- Oral supplementation will be required for the life of the animal.
- Daily dosing is required to maintain normal concentration of thyroid hormone.

- Excess medication can produce signs of hyperthyroidism: Increased thirst and urination, nervousness, weight loss, excessive panting, weakness, and increased appetite. If any of these signs are noticed, stop the medication and call your veterinarian.
- Follow-up blood tests may be required to ensure adequate hormone concentration.
- Certain drugs may decrease thyroid hormone concentration. Tell your veterinarian if your animal is currently taking any of these medications: Cortisone, aspirin, flunixin (Banamine), furosemide (Lasix), phenobarbital.

HYPERTHYROID DISEASE

Hyperthyroidism is the most commonly seen endocrine disorder in cats; however, it is seldom seen in the dog except as a result of neoplasia. The disease was first documented in the late 1970s to early 1980s, with incidence increasing steadily. The excess of both T_3 and T_4 results in a multisystemic disease seen primarily in older cats. Bilateral thyroid gland enlargement occurs in approximately 70% of cases and is the result of a functional thyroid adenoma. Thyroid carcinoma is rarely seen in the cat, comprising only 1% to 2% of all cases of hyperthyroidism.

CLINICAL SIGNS
- Middle age to older cat
- Weight loss
- Polyphagia
- Vomiting
- Increased appetite
- Tachycardia with or without murmurs
- Aggressive behavior
- Palpable enlarged thyroid
- Increased systolic blood pressure
- Blindness with retinal detachment

DIAGNOSIS
- Check for palpable enlarged thyroid.
- Test for elevated serum T_4 concentration.
- Perform serum chemistries to rule out other organ system failures that

may be present. Elevated ALT, alkaline phosphatase (ALP), and/or LDH are usually seen; elevated BUN and creatinine may be seen.
- Packed cell volume (PCV) is often in the high to normal range, stress leukogram.
- Check for abnormal thyroid radionuclide uptake imaging using either ^{131}I or ^{99m}Tc.

TREATMENT
- Control of excessive excretion of thyroid hormones can be accomplished by three methods. Choice of treatment depends on the severity of the disease, the age and physical status of the cat, and facilities available.

SURGERY
- Removal of the thyroid gland provides a cure for the disease, but it is important to preserve the parathyroid glands when removing thyroid tissue.

RADIOACTIVE IODINE-131
- This is the treatment of choice. Diseased tissue in the thyroid gland will take up larger amounts of radioactive ^{131}I than normal tissue. This uptake results in the destruction of the tissue, reducing thyroid hormone concentration. Cats should remain hospitalized until their wastes (especially urine) are below hazardous radiation levels (1 to 3 weeks).

ANTITHYROID DRUG THERAPY
- Antithyroid drugs inhibit the synthesis of thyroid hormone by disrupting the incorporation of iodine.
- Tapazole (methimazole): Initially administer 10 to 15 mg/day, adjusting the dose every 2 to 3 weeks (monitor T_4 concentration). Gradually increase the dose until the desired effect is achieved.

❶ TECH ALERT
Side effects include anorexia, vomiting, lethargy, and facial excoriation.
- Calcium ipodate: Administer 50 mg/kg/day PO.

INFORMATION FOR CLIENTS
- Surgery or radioactive iodine is the only cure for this disease.
- The cause of this disease is unknown.

- Medical management produces side effects in many cats. Report these to your veterinarian.
- Treatment to decrease thyroid hormone concentration may unmask concurrent diseases such as renal failure. This renal disease may be life threatening if not recognized.
- Concurrent diseases may need to be corrected before surgery.
- Bilateral removal of the thyroid glands may result in hypothyroidism, which will require daily treatment.
- All hyperthyroid patients should have blood pressure checked routinely. If Tapazole does not reduce blood pressure, then other antihypertensives should be added.

THE PANCREAS

DIABETES MELLITUS

Cells need glucose as a fuel. Through the processes of glycolysis, the citric acid cycle, electron transport, and oxidative phosphorylation, glucose is chemically converted into energy in the form of adenosine triphosphate (ATP), carbon dioxide, and water. It is therefore important for the body to regulate the concentration of glucose in circulation. Levels must be kept within certain limits to assure that adequate fuel is always available for energy production. The endocrine pancreas aids in this regulation; β-cells in the pancreatic islets (islets of Langerhans) produce the hormone insulin, which facilitates the entry of glucose into the cell for the process of glycolysis. Diabetes mellitus results when these β-cells stop producing insulin in adequate amounts or when the cells in specific body tissues become resistant to the action of insulin. The incidence of diabetes mellitus in the dog and cat is reported to be between 1 in 100 and 1 in 500. The cause of the disease is unknown, although chronic pancreatitis, immune-mediated disease, and hereditary predisposition have been suggested as possible causes.

Almost 100% of dogs and about 50% of cats will have *insulin-dependent diabetes (Type I)* at the time of presentation. As many as 50% of presenting cats will have *non–insulin-dependent diabetes (Type II),* which does not require insulin therapy.

Therapy for diabetes mellitus in most animals includes dietary regulation (usually a high-fiber diet) and daily insulin replacement. In non–insulin-dependent cats, drug therapy and diet restriction are somewhat successful in managing the disease.

The type of insulin chosen for therapy depends on the severity of the disease and patient needs. Treatment should be tailored to the species of animal involved. (Feline insulin most resembles beef insulin, and canine insulin resembles pork and human insulin.) Although it would be ideal to match the structure of each species' insulin, it is not easy to do this. Beef and pork insulin and their combinations have virtually disappeared from the market over the last 10 years; Humulin, human recombinant insulin, has taken their place as the most available insulin.

Diabetic patients whose sugar concentration remains uncontrolled may become *ketotic.* Cells begin to use fat as fuel for energy production, yielding *ketone bodies* that accumulate in the blood. Acidosis, dehydration, and electrolyte imbalances can occur as a result of ketosis.

CLINICAL SIGNS

NONKETOTIC DIABETES

- *Dogs:* 4 to 14 years of age, females twice as likely to be affected; *Cats:* All ages, with neutered males most affected
- Breeds predisposed to the disease: Poodles, Schnauzers, Keeshonds, Cairn Terriers, Dachshunds, Cocker Spaniels, and Beagles
- Polyuria (Pu)/polydipsia (Pd)
- Weight loss (especially in cats)
- Polyphagia
- Sudden cataract formation
- Dehydration
- Plantigrade posture in cats (walking on their hocks)

KETOTIC DIABETES

All of the above plus the following:

- Depression
- Weakness
- Tachypnea
- Vomiting
- Odor of acetone on the breath

DIAGNOSIS

- Evaluate clinical signs present in animal.
- Observe for documented fasting blood glucose concentration >200 mg/dl.

- Test urine for glycosuria.
- Complete serum chemistry to rule out other concurrent disease.

TREATMENT
DIETARY MANAGEMENT
- Restrict animal to a diet high in fiber and complex carbohydrates, such as Prescription Diet R/D or W/D (Hill's), Fit and Trim (Purina), or Science Diet Light (Hill's). This type of diet helps to avoid postprandial elevations of glucose and allows for better regulation of blood glucose concentration.

INSULIN THERAPY
- There are two types of insulin available, human (Humulin, Lilly) and beef/pork combination (Iletin I, Lilly). Most treatment regimens involve the use of neutral protamine Hagedorn (NPH, intermediate-acting) or Ultralente (long-acting) insulins.
- Recommended therapy doses:
  Dogs: Initially NPH insulin at a dose of 0.5 U/kg daily. Can be increased to twice daily if necessary.
  Cats: Ultralente insulin (Humulin, Lilly) at 1 to 3 U/cat daily or beef/pork lente insulin (Iletin, Lilly) at 1 to 3 U/cat twice daily.
- Insulin therapy should be monitored using improvement in clinical signs as a guide. Blood glucose concentration can be checked weekly to assist in adjusting the insulin dose. Animals that fail to regulate will require a glucose curve to adjust their insulin therapy.
- Serum fructose concentration can be monitored and will provide an evaluation of the average blood sugar concentration over a period of time. This value can be used to separate "stress hyperglycemia" from chronic hyperglycemia and is perhaps more valuable in regulating animals than spot checks on blood glucose.

INFORMATION FOR CLIENTS
- This disease will require life-long insulin replacement therapy.
- Insulin is given by injection.
- Because it is a protein molecule, insulin can be damaged by heat, rough handling, or chemicals. Refrigerate, mix gently, and avoid syringes that have been cleaned with soap or other cleaning agents.
- The formation of cataracts is the most common complication seen in diabetic animals. The process is irreversible once it occurs.
- Consistent feeding and exercise routines will make regulation easier.

- Animals will require periodic monitoring of blood glucose concentration for life.
- If untreated, the disease will progress and may lead to death.

Insulin Shock (Insulin Overdose)

Diabetic patients on insulin therapy will need to live a closely regulated lifestyle. Consistent feeding (both type and amount of food), exercise, and monitoring will make insulin regulation easier for the owner and safer for the pet. Patients who experience fluctuations in diet (do not eat consistent amounts or change foods frequently with loss of appetite) or who are allowed to exercise to excess can experience insulin shock. Exercise increases the need for glucose by body cells. This increased need uses up the exogenous insulin quickly, forcing glucose into the cells rapidly and dropping the blood concentration of glucose significantly. This rapid drop in glucose concentration in the blood results in a lack of glucose for the brain. Symptoms of weakness, restlessness, incoordination, seizures, and coma may develop. (These same symptoms may be seen in animals given an excessive dose of insulin by mistake.) The following schedule is recommended for feeding animals on insulin therapy:

- Monitor urine or blood glucose concentration at the same time each day.
- Base insulin dose on the current blood glucose measurements.
- Feed the animal one third of its total daily diet with insulin administration.
- Feed the remainder of the diet about 8 hours later (or at the time of measured peak insulin activity).
- Try to maintain a consistent daily exercise program—avoid excessive exercise. If the animal is expected to be more active than normal, give less insulin that day.

Owners should have a handy supply of sugar in case of insulin shock (Karo syrup, oral glucose solution or paste, treats). Owner should give these to the pet if any signs of insulin shock are present.

 TECH ALERT

Hyperglycemia is never acutely fatal, whereas hypoglycemia can be life threatening!

ADRENAL GLANDS

The adrenal glands are located dorsally and cranially to the kidneys, embedded in the perirenal fat (Fig. 4-3). They are comprised of two distinct regions, the

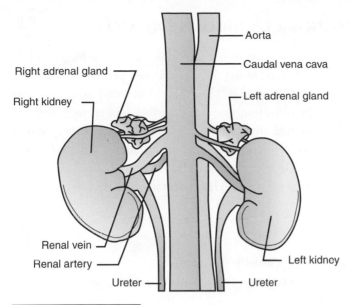

FIGURE 4-3.   Adrenal glands of the dog: ventral view. (From Colville T, Bassert JM: *Clinical anatomy and physiology for veterinary technicians*, St Louis, 2002, Mosby.)

medullary or *central area*, and the *cortical* or *outer area*, each of which produce distinct hormones.

The cortex produces three families of hormones: the *glucocorticoids*, the *mineralocorticoids*, and the *androgenic hormones (sex hormones)*. Glucocorticoids promote gluconeogenesis, suppress inflammation, suppress the immune system, and inhibit cartilage growth and development. They are not essential for life but are important for maintaining normal homeostasis. *Hyperadrenocorticism*, also known as *Cushing's syndrome*, occurs when excess glucocorticoids are produced by the adrenal gland.

Aldosterone is the principal mineralocorticoid. This hormone regulates electrolytes and has a potent effect on water metabolism within the body. Lack of this hormone is life threatening. *Hypoadrenocorticism*, or *Addison's disease*, is seen primarily in the dog and rarely in the cat.

The androgenic hormones produced by the adrenals are identical to those produced by the testicle. The small amount produced limits their effect on the animal.

The medullary area produces two hormones: *epinephrine* and *norepinephrine*. Both hormones affect the sympathetic nervous system and are involved in the "fight or flight" response.

The two most common diseases involving the adrenal glands are Cushing's syndrome and Addison's disease.

HYPOADRENOCORTICISM (ADDISON'S DISEASE)

Primary hypoadrenocorticism, most often classified as idiopathic, involves atrophy of the adrenal cortex resulting in a decreased production of both glucocorticoids and mineralocorticoids (loss of aldosterone is responsible for most of the clinical signs). An immune mechanism has been suggested for this disease. The disease is not common in dogs and is even more rare in cats. Other causes of hypoadrenocorticism include trauma, fungal infection, neoplasm, and hereditary tendencies (Standard Poodles and Labrador Retrievers). Excess amounts of the drug o,p'-DDD (mitotane) can also produce this disease.

CLINICAL SIGNS
- Middle age, female dogs (usually <7 years)
- Vague signs of depression, lethargy, weakness, anorexia, and weight loss
- Vomiting and diarrhea
- Pu/Pd
- Symptoms frequently wax and wane over time
- Bradycardia in about one third of all patients
- Dehydration

DIAGNOSIS
SERUM CHEMISTRY PANEL
- Test for a Na:K ratio of less than 27:1 (normal is between 27:2 and 40:1).
- Verify elevated BUN, creatinine, and calcium.
- Check for decreased blood sugar and albumin.
- Evaluate for acidosis.

ADRENOCORTICOTROPIC HORMONE (ACTH) STIMULATION TEST
- This test provides a definitive diagnosis of hypoadrenocorticism. ACTH gel (CortaGel 40, Savage Labs) or synthetic ACTH (Cortrosyn, Organon Pharm.) is given to the patient in the following doses:

  Gel: 2.2 U/kg IM with plasma cortisol samples at 0 and 120 minutes in dogs and 0, 60, and 120 minutes in cats.

  Synthetic: 0.25 mg/dog or 0.15 mg/cat IM with samples at 0 and 60 minutes in dogs and 0, 30, and 60 minutes in cats. Animals with hypoadrenocorticism typically have low resting cortisol concentration, which remains essentially unchanged after ACTH stimulation.

- *Endogenous ACTH concentration* testing must be done carefully, because ACTH is not stable over long periods of time. Concentrations will be elevated in dogs with primary (nonpituitary) hypoadrenocorticism.

❶ TECH ALERT

Vomiting dog with a high BUN and no kidney disease: Think Addison's disease.

TREATMENT

ACUTE CRISIS MANAGEMENT

- Normal saline is the fluid of choice for IV administration; give 44 to 88 ml/kg initially.
- Administer dexamethasone sodium phosphate 0.55 to 2.2 mg/kg IV, *or* prednisolone sodium succinate (Solu-delta-cortef) 4.4 to 22 mg/kg IV.
- Desoxycorticosterone pivalate (Percorten-V) 2.2 mg/kg IM or SQ, *or* fludrocortisone acetate (Florinef) 0.1 mg/4.5 kg daily PO can also be used.

CHRONIC MANAGEMENT

- Give oral glucocorticoids for 3 to 4 weeks, tapering dose gradually. Prednisolone or prednisone should be given in doses of 0.4 to 1.1 mg/kg/day, divided every 12 hours.
- Mineralocorticoid replacement requires Florinef 0.1 mg/4.5 kg/day divided every 12 hours.
- Monitor electrolytes, BUN/creatine, and clinical signs.

INFORMATION FOR CLIENTS

- Lack of mineralocorticoids is life threatening.
- Prognosis is excellent with medical treatment.
- Your pet will require periodic serum chemistry reevaluation.
- Most animals will need glucocorticoid supplementation in times of stress.
- In cases of trauma, surgery, or other stressful situations, make sure the treating veterinarian knows your pet suffers from hypoadrenocorticism so appropriate treatment can be provided.

HYPERADRENOCORTICISM (CANINE CUSHING'S SYNDROME)

Hyperadrenocorticism is rarely seen in the cat, but it is common in the dog. The term *canine Cushing's syndrome* is applied to any disease state that results in hypersecretion of cortisol. Excessive secretion of cortisol may result from a pituitary lesion (excess adrenocorticotropic hormone [ACTH]) or an adrenal tumor (excess cortisol). Hyperadrenocorticism frequently can be the result of overmedication with corticosteroids.

Pituitary-dependent disease (PDH) is seen most commonly in dogs weighing less than 20 kg. Breeds such as Poodles, Dachshunds, terriers, Beagles, and German Shepherds are affected. Boston Terriers and Boxers have been reported to be at increased risk of developing this disease. Abnormal cells within the pituitary gland secrete excessive amounts of ACTH; this results in hyperplasia of the adrenal glands, which is subsequently followed by oversecretion of cortisol. Although increased cortisol concentration usually serves to cause the pituitary to discontinue ACTH secretion, in these dogs the pituitary tissue fails to respond normally.

Functioning adrenal tumors secrete excessive amounts of cortisol independent of pituitary control. Dogs with this form of the disease are typically Toy Poodles, German Shepherds, Dachshunds, Labrador Retrievers, and some terrier breeds, with 45% to 50% weighing more than 20 kg.

Clinical signs of either type of Cushing's disease are the result of excess cortisol. They are usually slow to develop and often go unnoticed by the owner.

CLINICAL SIGNS
- Dog >6 years of age (60% to 65% are female)
- Pu/Pd
- Polyphagia
- Excessive panting
- Abdominal enlargement; obesity
- Muscle weakness, lethargy, lameness
- Bilateral, symmetrical alopecia, pruritus, pyoderma
- Calcinosis cutis (firm plaques of calcium under the skin)—infrequent
- Abnormal gonadal function—lack of estrus; soft, small testicles

DIAGNOSIS
SERUM CHEMISTRY PANEL ABNORMALITIES
- Increased ALP
- Increased ALT
- Increased cholesterol
- Increased blood glucose
- Decreased BUN
- Lipemia

URINE CORTISOL/CREATININE RATIOS
- Elevated
- Good for screening only

ACTH STIMULATION TEST
- Procedure is described under Addison's disease.
    PDH: 80% to 85% will be abnormal
    Adrenal: 20% to 40% may be normal

ⓘ TECH ALERT
May not be distinguishable from PDH and adrenal tumor

DEXAMETHASONE SUPPRESSION TEST
- In the normal animal, dexamethasone will suppress the pituitary secretion of ACTH, which, in turn, will decrease cortisol concentration within 2 to 3 hours and keep them suppressed for 8 to 24 hours.
- *Low Dose*
    PDH: No change in cortisol concentration at 8 hours postinjection
    Adrenal: No change in cortisol concentration

ⓘ TECH ALERT
Procedure: 0.01 mg/kg dexamethasone IV with samples at baseline (preinjection), 4 hours, and 8 hours postinjection
- *High Dose*
    0.1 mg/kg IV with samples at baseline and 8 hours postinjection
    PDH: Suppression seen at high doses; 75% to 80% of dogs with PDH will have 50% suppression of cortisol concentration.
    Adrenal: No suppression seen.

TREATMENT
SURGICAL REMOVAL
- One or both adrenal glands are removed.

MEDICAL MANAGEMENT
- The most frequent treatment choice is o,p'-DDD therapy (Lysodren, mitothane). The drug results in the necrosis of the zona fasciculata and zona reticularis; excessive doses will also affect the zona glomerulosa and reduce aldosterone concentration, producing Addison's disease.
- The initial therapy requires mitothane, 50 mg/kg/day in divided doses,

given after meals for 8 days. Monitor clinical signs for decrease in polyphagia and Pu/Pd. Repeat ACTH stimulation test every 7 to 10 days until cortisol concentrations are normal.

- Prednisone may be given during the loading dose regimen.
- Maintenance therapy requires the administration of o,p'-DDD at a dose of 25 mg/kg every 7 days.
- Other drugs used for treatment include the following:

    Ketoconazole: 5 mg/kg b.i.d. for 7 days. If no side effects appear, increase to 10 mg/kg b.i.d. for 14 days.

    L-Deprenyl: 2 mg/kg/day PO

INFORMATION FOR CLIENTS

- This is a serious disease.
- Animals will require life-long treatment.
- Periodic monitoring is required.
- Overdoses with o,p'-DDD are common.
- Clinical signs are identical to those in Addison's disease. Report any lethargy, weakness, vomiting, or diarrhea.
- Prognosis: Average life expectancy is about 20 to 30 months, with frequent recurrence of clinical symptoms.

DISEASES OF THE EYE five

Special structures exist in all animals that help them to survive in their environment. The special senses sight, hearing, smell, and taste are extensions of the central nervous system and are different from each other in their form and function. Problems involving sight and hearing are frequently seen in the dog and cat. This chapter focuses on ocular problems commonly seen in small animal practice. The topic of deafness may be found in Chapter 9, Diseases of the Nervous System.

The eye, made up of the globe and its accessory structures (Fig. 5-1), is perhaps the most highly developed of all the special senses. Its structure converts light into electrical impulses that travel to the brain and are interpreted as visual pictures.

The function of the eye depends on all components of the visual system functioning properly. Disruption of any of these components can result in abnormal vision for the animal. Although most of our pets can live quality lives with a loss of vision, proper diagnosis and quick treatment of eye problems is essential if sight is to be preserved.

Diseases of the eye may be divided into three main categories:
1. Those involving the accessory structures
   - Conjunctivitis
   - Epiphora
   - Keratoconjunctivitis sicca
   - "Cherry eye"
2. Those involving the structures within the globe
   - Corneal ulcers
   - Cataracts
   - Glaucoma
   - Uveitis
   - Trauma
3. Those involving the retina and the neural pathways
   - Progressive retinal atrophy

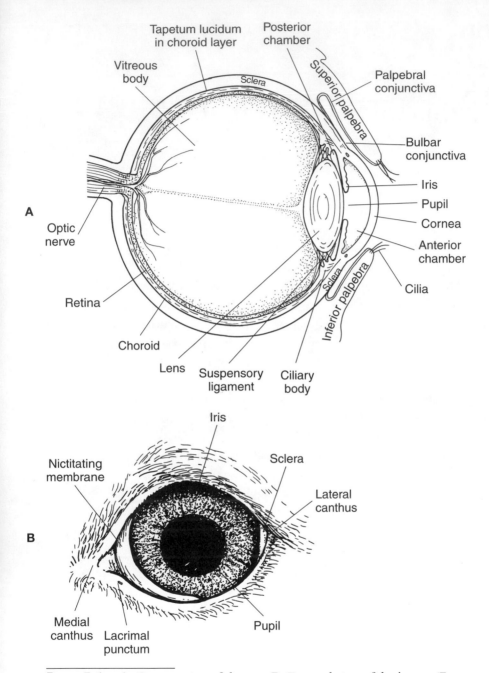

FIGURE 5-1. **A,** Cross-section of the eye. **B,** External view of dog's eye. (From McBride DF: *Learning veterinary terminology,* ed 2, St Louis, 2002, Mosby.)

DISEASES OF THE ACCESSORY STRUCTURES

Diseases involving the eyelids, conjunctiva, tear ducts, third eyelid, and the lacrimal glands may be included in this group. Trauma to or infection of these tissues is a common reason for small animals to be presented to the veterinary hospital. Typical presenting signs include red eyes, blepharospasm (squinting), and ocular discharge. Many eye problems present with similar signs; a thorough clinical examination is needed before a treatment plan can be formulated.

CONJUNCTIVITIS

Canine conjunctivitis, or inflammation of the conjunctiva, is rarely a primary disease process; therefore it is important for the veterinarian to discover the underlying cause to treat this condition effectively.

The conjunctiva is a highly vascular tissue. When injured, it responds by developing hyperemia (redness), chemosis (swelling), and ocular discharge. Dogs typically develop noninfectious conjunctivitis. Causes of noninfectious conjunctivitis in dogs include immune-mediated follicular conjunctivitis, allergic conjunctivitis (atopy), and anatomic conjunctivitis (ectropion/entropion). Bacterial conjunctivitis can develop in the dog as a result of the disruption of normal tear production, injury, or foreign bodies.

Feline conjunctivitis is primarily infectious. Feline herpes virus (FHV) is the most common cause of bilateral conjunctivitis in young kittens and is typically seen in conjunction with upper respiratory tract symptoms. FHV-1 virus replicates best in epithelial tissue that is slightly cooler than body temperature and therefore tends to infect the superficial epithelial tissues of the nasal, oral, and conjunctival regions.

Calici virus may also cause a mild conjunctivitis in cats. *Chlamydia psittaci* infection may present as a unilateral problem with marked chemosis in some cats. Mycoplasmas have also been isolated from cases of feline conjunctivitis.

CLINICAL SIGNS
- Chemosis
- Hyperemia
- Ocular discharge (serous or purulent)
- Presence or absence of other signs of upper respiratory tract disease

DIAGNOSIS
- A complete physical examination is necessary to diagnose the primary disease.

- A thorough visual examination of the conjunctiva must be conducted to rule out foreign bodies or the presence of follicles.
- The Schirmer tear test is useful in recurrent cases.
- Conjunctival scraping may need to be performed, including cytology, culture, and sensitivity.

TREATMENT
- Treat to resolve the underlying systemic disease.
- Topical antibiotic ointments can be used, including:
    Neomycin/bacitracin/polymyxin B ointment: 2 to 4 times daily (general cases)
    Gentamycin ophthalmic ointment: 2 to 4 times daily for bacterial infections
    Antibiotic ointment with cortisone for cases involving follicular or atopic conjunctivitis
- Nonsteroidal ointments and solutions may be necessary, including:
    Ketorolac tromethamine 0.5%: 4 times daily for allergic conjunctivitis
    Lodoxamide tromethamine 0.1%: 4 times daily for allergic conjunctivitis
- Keep eyes clear of dried exudate by using warm water and a cloth or a cotton ball.
- For viral conjunctivitis in cats, the following can be used:
    Idoxuridine (IDU, Stoxil) 0.5%, q 4 to 5 h
    Adenine arabinoside (Vir-A) 3%, 1 drop q 2 h

INFORMATION FOR CLIENTS
- Prevent irritation of the conjunctiva in dogs by not allowing them to ride with their heads out of car windows.
- Keep dried ocular discharge from accumulating in the medial canthus of the eye. Keep the area clean and dry. Remove excess hair that may trap exudate.
- Vaccinate kittens against respiratory viral disease as per your veterinarian's schedule.
- When using ophthalmic medications, make sure not to touch the tip of the applicator to the eye; this will contaminate the container.
- Ointments provide longer tissue contact than do solutions.
- Ophthalmic preparations must be applied frequently to be effective.
- Ask your technician to demonstrate the proper method for administering eye ointments (Fig. 5-2).

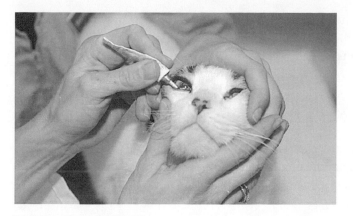

Figure 5-2. Placing eye ointment on the lower palpebral border in a cat. (From McCurnin DM, Bassert JM: *Clinical textbook for veterinary technicians,* ed 5, St Louis, 2002, WB Saunders.)

- Discard any unused eye medications as soon as treatment is no longer needed. Do not save them for future use!

Epiphora

Epiphora, an overflow of tears, may be the result of overproduction of tears or faulty drainage by the lacrimal system. Overproduction of tears is always the result of ocular pain or irritation. Faulty functioning of the lacrimal drainage system may occur for several reasons, including blockage of the lacrimal duct by swelling or inflammatory cells, imperforate puncta, or trauma.

Brachycephalic dogs and cats have large globes in shallow orbits leaving little room for the accumulation of tears. Subsequently, tears spill out onto the face. Accumulations of hair or face folds may wick the tears onto the face in some animals. An entropion or ectropion may also result in faulty drainage of tears.

Surgical correction of lid position is the treatment of choice in animals having entropion or ectropion. Keeping the facial hair cut shorter may also be beneficial. Obstruction of the lacrimal puncta may occur in animals as a result of inflammation, the presence of foreign bodies, or accumulation of debris. Cocker Spaniels and Poodles typically have imperforate puncta (no opening to provide drainage). Many times the obstruction can be removed by flushing the nasolacrimal ducts or surgically removing the tissue covering the puncta.

Facial hair or cilia originating from the meibomian glands of the lid may rub against the cornea, creating irritation and, often, corneal ulceration. Epiphora then results as a reflex against the pain created by the irritation. Treatment includes removal of the cilia or shortening of the facial hair and topical therapy.

CLINICAL SIGNS
- "Watering" of the eye—may be acute or chronic
- Wet facial hair in the medial canthus
- Secondary bacterial infection of the skin underlying the hair at the medial canthus
- Discoloration of the facial hair at the medial canthus

DIAGNOSIS
- Perform a complete eye examination to find the source of pain.
- Apply fluorescein dye to the eye. Dye that exits the nares indicates a patent nasolacrimal system in most patients.
- Dacryocystorhinography can be performed in recurring cases.

TREATMENT
- Treat the primary cause of ocular pain and irritation.
- Flush the lacrimal ducts to remove any obstructions (Fig. 5-3).
- Surgically open imperforate puncta.
- Apply a topical antibiotic ointment for 7 to 10 days.
- Keep facial hair trimmed to prevent contact with the cornea.

INFORMATION FOR CLIENTS
- Keep facial hair trimmed in the eye area to prevent wicking of tears and accumulation of debris in the corner of the eye.
- The red stain seen on the hair of white or light colored dogs is not blood but a pigment contained in the tears. It will not hurt the dog.
- In some breeds, epiphora may be a life-long problem requiring continual maintenance.

EYELID DISEASES

The eyelids are important for ocular health. They protect the globe, help to remove debris from the eye, shade the eye during sleep, and spread lubricating

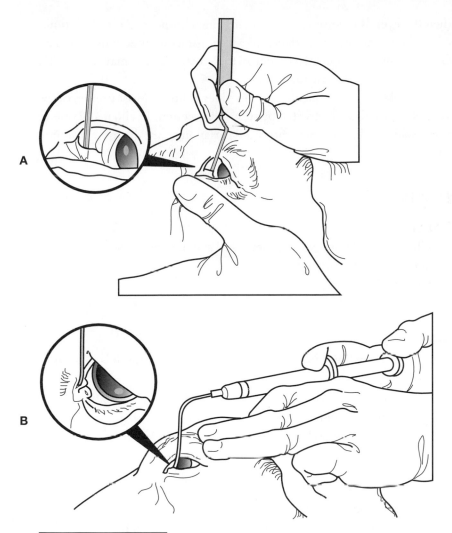

FIGURE 5-3. **A,** Dilating puncta of nasolacrimal duct with blunt metal probe.
B, Flushing nasolacrimal duct.

secretions over the eye. Eyelashes project from the border of each lid. At the base of each lash is a sebaceous gland, which produces a lubricating fluid for the hair follicles (glands of Zeis or meibomian glands).

An abscess of the sebaceous gland is called a *hordeolum* and is usually the result of a staphylococcal infection. When the inflammation involves the meibomian glands and granuloma formation occurs, it is called a *chalazion*. Therapy for both of these swellings includes warm compresses, manual expression, topical antibiotic ointment, and possibly surgical curettage.

When the eyelids themselves become inflamed, *blepharitis* results. Etiologies include bacterial infections *(Staphylococcus)*, parasitic infections *(Demodex, Notoedres)*, and mycotic infections (dermatophytes). Atopy may frequently present with inflamed and pruritic eyelids.

Eyelid neoplasms are frequently seen in older animals. Most tumors of the eyelids are benign and can be treated by surgical resection. Eyelid neoplasms in the cat are usually malignant. Squamous cell carcinomas are the most common type of tumor.

BLEPHARITIS

CLINICAL SIGNS
- Swelling at the lid margin or generalized swelling of the lid
- Periocular pruritus
- Periocular alopecia
- Rubbing of the eyes

DIAGNOSIS
- Careful examination must be made of the eyes and the lids. This may require magnification.
- Skin scraping of periorbital area is often necessary.
- Fungal cultures should be obtained.
- Bacterial cultures should be obtained.

TREATMENT
- Warm compresses should be applied to reduce swelling.
- Express hordeolum or remove chalazion.
- Topical antibiotic ointments or systemic antibiotics can be applied:
    Chloramphenicol (ophthalmic)
    Gentamycin (ophthalmic ointment or drops)
    Tetracycline (ophthalmic)
    Neobacimyx
    Mycitracin
    Optiprime
    Trioptics
    Neo-Predef
- Corticosteroid: Prednisolone 1.1 mg/kg b.i.d. 10 to 14 days then gradually reduce dose

- Mycotic: Topical antifungal solutions such as Conofite or Tresaderm (before you apply these around the eye, place protective ointment into the eye)

INFORMATION FOR CLIENTS

- Warm packs applied to the swollen, painful eyelids may provide relief for the patient. Use a cotton ball soaked in warm water, soak a cloth in warm water and ring well to remove excess water, or use a hot pack *warmed* in the microwave (take care not to make it too hot).
- Remove exudate from the corners of the eye several times daily using a soft, wet cloth or cotton ball.

ENTROPION AND ECTROPION

These defects (entropion and ectropion) involve eyelids that either roll in against the cornea (entropion) or roll outward, exposing the cornea (ectropion). In either case, the lids are incapable of performing their protective functions for the eye and disease may result.

Entropion is common in dogs, but less common in cats. There are three main forms of the defect: congenital (inherited), acquired nonspastic, and acquired spastic. The congenital form includes those breeds predisposed to entropion owing to large orbits with deep-set eyes, which provide inadequate lid support. The lid droops over the lower orbital rim and inverts. Collies, Great Danes, Irish Setters, Doberman Pinschers, Golden Retrievers, Rottweilers, and Weimaraners are breeds that exhibit congenital entropion.

Several breeds are predisposed to poor muscular development involving the ocular muscles. Chesapeake Bay Retrievers, Labrador Retrievers, Chow Chows, and Samoyeds may exhibit this condition, although it is not well documented. A great number of breeds are predisposed to entropion from primary lid deformities.

The etiology of acquired nonspastic entropion is usually surgical or traumatic, resulting in scarring of the lid with contraction. This causes the lid to turn inward toward the globe. The third form of entropion is acquired spastic and is the most commonly observed form in cats. This form of entropion usually occurs secondary to painful corneal lesions and/or conjunctival inflammation.

Ectropion is the reverse of entropion. In this condition, the lid is excessive and droops outward. Ectropion is a natural breed characteristic in Basset

Hounds, Bloodhounds, Cocker/Cumber Spaniels, English Bulldogs, and Saint Bernards. In these animals it is usually asymptomatic. In any breed, however— even the ones listed—ectropion can develop clinical symptoms. Acquired ectropion can form secondary to muscular disease in senile dogs that lose muscle tone and in dogs that have had overcorrection of an entropion.

CLINICAL SIGNS
ENTROPION
- Rolling inward of the lid margin(s)
- Epiphora
- Chemosis
- Conjunctival erythema, conjunctivitis
- Blepharospasm
- Pain
- Presence or absence of corneal ulceration
- Photophobia

ECTROPION
- Lid eversion
- Conjunctivitis
- Epiphora
- Keratitis, usually from exposure
- Purulent exudate

DIAGNOSIS
- Observe the lids and their interaction with the globe.
- Complete an evaluation of other structures of the eye, especially the cornea, conjunctiva, and lid margins.
- The evaluation of lid inversion or eversion should be done while the patient is awake to prevent overcorrection or undercorrection of the defect.

TREATMENT
ENTROPION
- Surgical correction is suggested:
  - Temporary vertical mattress suture placement to evert the eye (young animals)
  - Lateral canthoplasty to shorten the lid

Hotz-Celsus procedure: An elliptical piece of tissue is removed from under the eye to evert the lid into a normal position.

ECTROPION

- Surgical correction is recommended if clinical signs are present:
    V plasty procedure to shorten the lid
    Lateral blepharoplasty
    V-Y plasty if scar tissue has contracted the lid in an everted position

INFORMATION FOR CLIENTS

- You may want to avoid purchasing breeds predisposed to entropion or ectropion.
- Carefully examine puppies for these defects before purchasing them. Dogs usually do not "outgrow" these conditions.
- Correction of these defects will provide normal lid function and save the globe from damage by preventing overexposure to the environment and by reducing contact with the lid margins.

HYPERTROPHY OF NICTITANS GLAND (CHERRY EYE)

The nictitating membrane (third eyelid) is important as a protective structure. It assists in spreading the precorneal tear film and covers the eye to protect it from injury. It also produces about 50% of the lacrimal fluid.

The membrane is composed of a T-shaped cartilaginous skeleton embedded in the superficial gland of the third eyelid. The tissue undergoes what has been described as passive forward displacement when the eye is withdrawn into the orbit. This action results in prolapse of the third eyelid.

Hypertrophy of the gland (cherry eye) occurs only in the dog. The etiology is unknown; however, there is a breed predisposition (Basset Hound, Beagle, Boston Terrier, Cocker Spaniel). When this condition is present, the medial canthus is filled with the red, swollen nictating membrane, which resembles a small cherry. This is usually seen in young dogs (<2 years). When the condition occurs in older animals and in cats, the cause is usually related to neoplasia of the tissue comprising the third eyelid.

CLINICAL SIGNS

- Reddened enlargement of tissue in the medial canthus of the eye
- Mild irritation, usually no pain

- Epiphora
- Presence or absence of conjunctival irritation

DIAGNOSIS
- Clinical signs
- Predisposed breed
- Tumor has been ruled out in older dogs and cats

TREATMENT
- Surgical replacement of the gland using tack down procedures
- *Avoid* excision of the gland, as it will predispose the animal to keratoconjunctivitis sicca (KCS) later in life. Excision should only be used in cases of neoplasia of the gland.

INFORMATION FOR CLIENTS
- Surgery is the only method of correction.
- Without surgery, the animal may suffer corneal damage that may affect eyesight.

DISEASES OF THE EYE

GLAUCOMA

The eyeball represents a relatively closed system housed in a bony orbit. An increase in the contents of the globe results in increased intraocular pressure (IOP) because expansion is limited. In the normal eye, the production of aqueous fluid is equal to the amount leaving the eye and the IOP remains fairly constant. If more aqueous fluid is produced than leaves the eye, glaucoma results.

Normal canine and feline IOP ranges from 12 to 22 mm Hg. Values greater than 30 mm Hg are diagnostic for glaucoma. Most canine glaucoma cases result from decreased outflow of aqueous fluid as opposed to increased production. IOP may be measured by using a Schiotz tonometer or a Tonopen.

Glaucoma may be primary or secondary. Primary glaucoma is an inherited defect affecting both eyes. Cocker Spaniels, Basset Hounds, and Chow Chows are predisposed to primary glaucoma. Secondary glaucoma results from obstruction of the drainage angles secondary to another disease process such as a neoplasm, uveitis, lens luxation, or hemorrhage.

Glaucoma may also be acute or chronic. Acute development of severely elevated IOP (>60 mm Hg) can produce blindness within hours owing to disruption of retinal ganglion cells and retinal circulation. The goal of treatment is to decrease IOP rapidly to prevent permanent injury.

Sustained IOP in chronic glaucoma produces a painful, blind eye, which is unresponsive to medical therapy. Salvage procedures to make the pet more comfortable are the only recommended treatments.

CLINICAL SIGNS

Acute

- Ocular pain
- Conjunctival and episcleral injection (vascular congestion)
- Diffuse corneal edema
- Dilated pupil, unresponsive or sluggish to light
- Animal may or may not be blind on presentation.

Chronic

- Buphthalmus (enlarged globe)
- Corneal striae
- Optic disk cupping
- Pain
- Blindness

DIAGNOSIS

- Measured IOP >30 mm Hg
- Clinical signs
- Rule out (R/O) lens luxation as cause.

TREATMENT

Acute

 TECH ALERT

This is a true emergency.

- Latanoprost (Xalatan 0.005%): 1 drop q 24 h to facilitate aqueous outflow
- IV mannitol: 1 to 1.5 g/kg slowly over 20 to 30 min
- Oral dichlorphenamide (Daranide, Merck): 10 to 15 mg/kg q 8 h PO; decreases aqueous humor production

- Topical pilocarpine (pilocarpine 2%): Instill into the eye q 6 h. Used to increase aqueous outflow.
- Timolol 0.5% (Timoptic, Merck) can be used in combination with carbonic anhydrase inhibitors like Daranide.
- Treatment may include one or more of the above drugs depending on the clinical presentation and personal experience.

SURGICAL

- Procedures that decrease aqueous production by destroying part of the ciliary body:
    Transscleral cryosurgery
    Laser cyclophotocoagulation

❶ TECH ALERT

Both of these may cause postoperative increases in IOP that may result in permanent blindness. The laser method seems to produce better results with fewer side effects.

- Procedures that increase outflow of aqueous fluid: These are usually expensive and require referral to a specialty practice.

CHRONIC

- For a blind, painful eye, surgery is the treatment of choice to relieve the pain.
    Enucleation
    Intraocular evisceration with an implant
    Ciliary ablation using gentamycin intravitreal injection

INFORMATION FOR CLIENTS

- Have your pet examined immediately when signs of a red, swollen, painful eye occur. This may be a true emergency, and vision can be quickly lost if treatment is postponed.
- This condition will require life-long treatment.
- The disease is progressive.
- Even with proper treatment, vision may be lost in the affected eye as the disease progresses.
- Blind animals can live happy, comfortable lives. Their extra senses allow them to adjust well to the loss of sight.

- Avoid moving or changing a blind pet's environment too rapidly. They need time to adjust.
- Breeds that are predisposed to glaucoma include Cocker Spaniels, Basset Hounds, Miniature Poodles, Boston Terriers, Dalmatians, Arctic breeds, and Beagles.
- Enucleation (removal of the affected eye) will relieve the severe pain that results from glaucoma and will greatly improve the animal's quality of life.

ULCERATIVE KERATITIS (CORNEAL ULCERS)

The cornea is the "window" of the eye and is composed of four layers: the epithelium, the stroma, Descemet's membrane, and the endothelium. The epithelial covering provides a barrier to microorganisms entering the eye. A corneal ulcer is a full-thickness loss of corneal epithelium that exposes the underlying stroma. Causes of ulceration include trauma, chemicals, foreign objects, diseases such as keratoconjunctivitis sicca, and conformational abnormalities. In cats, herpes virus can directly invade the corneal epithelium and produce ulceration.

Patients usually present with pain, epiphora, blepharospasm, and conjunctival hyperemia. Diagnosis involves using fluorescein dye, which is absorbed well by the corneal stroma but not by intact corneal epithelium. The ulcerated area will fluoresce green when exposed to light with a cobalt blue filter.

Corneal epithelium will heal rapidly as cells divide and migrate. Treatment of uncomplicated ulcers includes application of topical atropine ointment to decrease pain and a topical antibiotic ointment. In most cases, ulcers will heal within several days. If the ulcers do not heal, alternative methods of treatment should be considered.

Distichiasis (hairs from the meibomian glands on the inner lid surface), ectopic cilia, and trichiasis (normal hairs that rub on the cornea) are frequent causes of ulcers in some breeds. A thorough examination of the eyelids is required (under magnification) to find these culprits.

Infected ulcers may also heal slowly. A culture and sensitivity should be obtained if infection is suspected.

Indolent ulcers (Boxer ulcers) fail to heal even after weeks of therapy. The epithelium is usually undermined at the edge of the ulcer, preventing migration of healing tissue across the lesion. Treatment may involve a grid keratectomy or a superficial keratectomy.

CLINICAL SIGNS
- Epiphora
- Blepharospasm
- Hyperemia of conjunctiva

DIAGNOSIS
- Fluorescein dye applied to the cornea will have a green fluorescence under cobalt blue light if epithelium is not intact.
- Complete a thorough eye examination—look for aberrant cilia/hairs and foreign material. Be sure to look under the third eyelid.
- Perform a culture and sensitivity if you suspect an infectious agent.

TREATMENT
- Topical atropine 1% ointment can be used to decrease pain and blepharospasm.
- Topical broad-spectrum antibiotic ophthalmic ointment can be used 4 to 6 times daily.
- Surgery is another option.
    Grid keratotomy (does not seem to improve healing time in cats)
    Superficial keratotomy
    Eyelid flaps
    Conjunctival flaps
    Contact lenses
- Serum: Prepare patient serum from a blood sample. Apply 1 drop into the eye every 2 to 4 hours daily. Recheck in 24 to 48 hours for healing.

INFORMATION FOR CLIENTS
- Most ulcers will heal quickly with treatment.
- Avoid using old medications you may have in the refrigerator to treat a red, watering eye.
- Medications containing cortisone will retard healing and make the ulcer worse.
- Discard any ophthalmic medications after the prescribed period of use.
- Ulcers that involve dissolution of the corneal epithelium, indolent ulcers, or ulcers that involve Descemet's membrane are serious and will require aggressive treatment.
- When using ophthalmic medications, take care not to touch the eye or the tissue around the eye with the end of the medicine container. This will result in contamination of the medication.

- Frequent rechecks by your veterinarian will be necessary to follow the healing of your pet's ulcer.

Chronic Superficial Keratitis (Pannus)

The term *pannus* is used to describe superficial corneal vascularization and infiltration of granulation tissue. The disease is progressive, bilateral, and degenerative and potentially can result in blindness. Lesions typically begin at the limbus and progressively enlarge to involve the entire cornea. The etiology is thought to be immune-mediated, and middle-age animals living at elevations greater than 5000 feet are most susceptible. Increased levels of ultraviolet light also increase incidence. Breeds commonly associated with the development of pannus include the German Shepherd, Belgian Tervuren, Border Collie, Greyhound, and Siberian Husky. Lesions typically involve infiltration of the cornea with lymphocytes and plasma cells. Treatment is life-long and is aimed at lesion regression and control.

CLINICAL SIGNS
- Breed predisposed to disease with opaque lesion beginning at the limbus and extending into the cornea (may be pink or tan)

DIAGNOSIS
- Perform a corneal scraping. Positive cytology will show lymphocytic-plasmocytic infiltrate.
- Complete a thorough eye examination to rule out KCS, corneal ulcers, or other pathologies.

TREATMENT
- Antiinflammatory agents for the life of the patient include:
  - Topical cyclosporine A (Optimune) q.i.d.
  - 1% prednisolone acetate (AK-Tate)
  - 1% prednisolone sodium phosphate (AK-Pred)
  - 0.1% dexamethasone ophthalmic (AK-Dex)
- Subconjunctival injection may be necessary: Triamcinolone acetonide (Vetalog) 0.1 ml/2 wk or methylprednisolone acetate (DepoMedrol): g/ml; 0.2 ml/3 wk
- Cryosurgery with liquid nitrogen is also an option.
- Superficial keratectomy will be required if all other treatments fail and loss of vision occurs.

INFORMATION FOR CLIENTS

- There is no cure for pannus. Treatment to maintain regression of the lesion will be life-long.
- If treatment is inconsistent or discontinued, the lesion will return and continue to expand.
- Dogs living at higher altitudes and exposed to ultraviolet radiation (sunlight) are at greater risk of developing this disease.

KERATOCONJUNCTIVITIS SICCA (KCS)

Continuous production and distribution of tears are necessary for maintaining a healthy cornea. Tears clean, lubricate, nourish, reduce bacteria, and aid in healing. The tear film is composed of three layers. The lipid layer is secreted by the meibomian glands and aids in tear distribution. The aqueous layer, which is produced by the lacrimal glands and makes up the bulk of tear volume, contains immunoglobulins, enzymes, glucose, proteins, ions, and salts. The mucous, or innermost, layer is secreted by the conjunctival goblet cells and aids in the adhesion of the tear layer to the corneal surface.

Dogs and cats have two lacrimal glands, one located in the lateral superior orbit and one at the base of the third eyelid. Approximately 70% of the total tear volume is produced by the orbital gland. The nictitans is responsible for the remaining 30% of production. Loss of both glands (atrophy) produces KCS.

Causes of KCS include viral infections, drug-related toxicities, immune-mediated disease, inflammation, breed predisposition, and congenital anomalies. Most cases are idiopathic, but the disease tends to occur in older animals (usually >7 years). The disease is more common in neutered animals because loss of sex hormones decreases tear production. Diagnosis requires a complete medical history and a comprehensive physical examination. Treatment is aimed at restoring tear production and controlling secondary infections.

CLINICAL SIGNS

- Recurrent conjunctivitis, corneal ulcers, keratitis
- Cornea and conjunctiva appear dull, dry, and irregular
- Tenacious mucoid ocular discharge on lid margins and in the medial canthus
- Blepharospasm
- Crusty nares

DIAGNOSIS

- Schirmer tear test: Values <15 mm/min on repeat testing (normal values: canine, 15 to 25 mm/min; feline, 11 to 23 mm/min)
- Corneal fluorescein staining to reveal ulcers

TREATMENT

- Tear stimulation: Cyclosporine (Optimmune), apply to eye every 8 hours; oral pilocarpine 2%, 1 to 2 drops/9 kg BW in food twice daily (side effects include salivation, vomiting, diarrhea, and bradycardia)
- Topical artificial tear ointments:
    Duo-lube (B&L)
    Hypo Tears (IOLab)
    Lacri-lube (Allergan)

⚠ TECH ALERT

Ointments remain in contact with the cornea longer than solutions and require less frequent applications.

- Topical antibiotic ointments (broad spectrum); neomycin-bacitracin-polymyxin
- *Avoid* atropine, contact lenses, topical anesthetics, and corticosteroids if ulceration is present.
- Surgery: If all other medical treatments are unsuccessful—parotid duct transposition

INFORMATION FOR CLIENTS

- The prognosis for resolution is guarded.
- Treatment will need to continue for the life of the animal.
- About 15% to 20% of patients may exhibit remission with return of tear production.
- Failure to treat these animals will result in blindness.

CATARACTS

The most common disease involving the lens is cataract formation. A cataract may be defined as an opacity of the lens sufficient to cause a reduction in visual function. Cataracts are a frequent cause of blindness in the dog but also are seen occasionally in the cat. Most cataracts in the dog are inherited, but cataracts may also occur secondary to diabetes mellitus, hypocalcemia, trauma, nutritional deficiencies, electric shock, uveitis, or lens luxation.

Cataracts must be differentiated from senile nuclear (lenticular) sclerosis, a normal change in aging animals. Aging cells within the lens become dehydrated and overlap each other, producing a central change in the reflection of light. The lens may appear grey and opaque; however, with lenticular sclerosis, vision is maintained, and the ocular fundus is visible by ophthalmoscopy.

Surgical removal of a primary cataract is the only means of treatment and should be considered if the animal has bilateral cataracts with significantly impaired vision or the animal is unable to maintain a normal lifestyle. Before surgery it is important to establish the integrity of the retina and visual pathways. Removal of a cataract is unnecessary if vision has been lost to concurrent retinal or optic nerve disease. The electroretinogram provides the most reliable criteria for retinal evaluation; however, it is limited to use in referral centers. If visual pathways are intact, cataract surgery can successfully restore the animal's sight.

Cataracts that result secondary to other disease states will require medical management of those diseases before surgical removal.

CLINICAL SIGNS
- Progressive loss of vision
- Opaque pupillary opening (usually noticed by owner)
- Signs related to systemic diseases such as diabetes mellitus or hypocalcemia

DIAGNOSIS
- Perform a complete ophthalmologic examination.
- Assess vision based on completion of an obstacle course, lack of menace response, and failure to track visual responses (use cotton balls).
- Pupillary light response (PLR) is usually normal.
- Test serum chemistries to rule out concurrent systemic disease.
- Electroretinogram should be used to rule out retinal degeneration or optic nerve disease.

TREATMENT
- Surgical removal of the cataract is necessary.
- Treatment of any other disease that may result in the formation of the cataract must be completed first.

INFORMATION FOR CLIENTS
- Most cataracts are inherited, so affected animals should not be used for breeding.
- Certain breeds are prone to cataract and/or retinal degeneration.
- Many animals can have quality lives even with bilateral cataracts.
- To decrease the chance of postoperative complications, most surgeons will remove only one cataract.
- Surgery will require referral to a veterinary ophthalmologist with special training; this will be expensive.
- Function of the visual pathway must be ensured before surgery.

ANTERIOR UVEITIS

The uvea is the pigmented vascular tunic located between the fibrous and nervous tunics. It includes the iris, the ciliary body, and the choroid. Inflammation of this tissue is known as uveitis.

Anterior uveitis may have several etiologies: trauma, extension of local infections, foreign bodies, neoplasm, or thermal trauma. Bacterial, viral, and mycotic diseases may undergo hematogenous spread to the uvea. Parasites and protozoa also may affect the tissue. Some cases may be immune-mediated. Whatever the etiology, the symptoms will be similar; prompt treatment will be needed to prevent permanent damage to the eye.

CLINICAL SIGNS
- Epiphora
- Blepharospasm
- Photophobia
- Presence or absence of vision defects
- Corneal edema (cornea will be gray/white)
- Chemosis of the conjunctiva
- Scleral injection
- Prolapsed third eyelid
- Pain
- Change in color of the iris if chronic

DIAGNOSIS
- Clinical signs
- History

- CBC, serum chemistries to rule out systemic disease
- Immunology screening panel to rule out brucellosis, toxoplasmosis, blastomycosis, cryptococcus, leptospirosis, ICH, FIP, and FeLV
- Radiography or ultrasound examination of the eye
- Tonometry: IOP may be low (4 to 8 mm Hg) or elevated (>27 mm Hg)

TREATMENT
- Identify and eliminate the immediate cause of the uveitis if possible.
- Control inflammation.
    Topical steroids: Dexamethasone ophthalmic ointment q 4 to 6 h
    Banamine: IV in dogs only: 0.25 mg/kg s.i.d.

ⓘ TECH ALERT
Do not use banamine in dogs taking aspirin.
   Aspirin: 1 g/10 kg t.i.d. in dogs; 1 g/10 kg b.i.d. in cats

- Atropine 1% ophthalmic ointment helps to restore the integrity of vascular permeability and prevent adhesions of the lens to the iris by dilating the pupil. Use every 4 hours until dilated, then decrease to maintain mydriasis (dilation).

INFORMATION FOR CLIENTS
- The prognosis is excellent for uncomplicated cases.
- Most of the diseases that can result in secondary anterior uveitis are extremely serious and may not be curable.
- Diagnosis and treatment of the initial disease may be costly and prolonged.
- Without treatment, vision will eventually be lost.

PROGRESSIVE RETINAL ATROPHY (PRA)

The inner posterior portion of the eye is composed of the retina, the neural tunic of the eyeball where the visual pathway begins. Located within the optic disk, the optic nerve exits each eye and extends toward the brain. Arteries and veins fan out from the nerve to nourish the anterior surface of the retina. Within the retina are the photoreceptor cells (rods and cones) that are responsible for light sensing. Rods are functional for black-and-white vision and low light situations, whereas the cones are bright light receptors and are responsible for color vision. The retina must be functioning normally for vision to occur.

Progressive retinal atrophy (PRA) is the term used to describe a group of hereditary retinal disorders seen in many breeds of dogs. The disease is common in Toy Poodles, Miniature Poodles, Golden Retrievers, Irish Setters, Cocker Spaniels, Miniature Schnauzers, Collies, Samoyed, Gordon Setters, and Norwegian Elkhounds. Inheritance has been shown to be by an autosomal recessive gene in several of these breeds. There is no sex predilection. Signs of the disease can be detected in some breeds as early as 6 months old (Irish Setter, Collie) and in others by middle age (Poodles). Clinical signs are usually slow to develop; a loss of night or low light vision occurs first. As the disease progresses, day vision may be affected. Cataracts often develop in the affected eye. Diagnosis is through a complete ophthalmoscopic examination and an electroretinogram (ERG). The end-stage lesions are those of retinal thinning with retinal nerve atrophy and vascular attenuation. There is no cure or treatment.

Retinal atrophy does occur in cats but not as frequently as in dogs. Central retinal degeneration in the feline is related to taurine-deficient diet.

CLINICAL SIGNS
- Defective night vision
- Slowly progressive loss of day vision
- Cataract formation

DIAGNOSIS
- Perform complete blood count and serum chemistries to rule out other causes of cataracts and/or loss of vision.
- Ophthalmological examination of the retina early on will reveal a gray, granular appearance of the peripheral tapetal retina. Under bright light, the area may appear hyperreflective. As the disease progresses, the retina will become thinner, resulting in increased reflectivity. End-stage lesions will include severe vascular attenuation and optic nerve atrophy.
- ERG is abnormal.

TREATMENT
- None

INFORMATION FOR CLIENTS
- This is an inherited disease. Avoid buying breeds affected with this defect unless the animal has had a complete eye examination by a board-

certified veterinary ophthalmologist and the animal is certified free of the disease.

- Blind animals seem to adapt well to their familiar environment and will have trouble only when placed in strange surroundings.
- Cats must be fed a taurine-rich diet to avoid retinal degeneration.

Hematologic and Immunologic Diseases six

Immune-mediated and hematologic disorders are commonly seen in veterinary practice. Although these diseases may be interrelated in some cases, this chapter discusses the most important diseases as individual entities. The technician is referred to a veterinary hematology text for review of the sequence of erythropoiesis and the function of the immune system. You may also refer to Chapter 1. Knowledge of hematology and the functions of the immune system will assist the student in understanding these diseases.

ERYTHROCYTE DISORDERS

Erythrocyte disorders are frequently diagnosed in the dog and cat and may be associated with either decreased production, increased destruction, or inappropriate loss of red blood cells (hemorrhage). Included in this category of disorders are anemias, hemorrhage, and neoplasia.

Anemia is one of the most common laboratory findings encountered in veterinary medicine and is usually secondary to a primary disorder elsewhere in the body. The major causes of anemia are varied and include hemorrhage, hemolysis, blood parasites, iron deficiencies, immune-mediated disease, and toxins.

A systematic diagnostic approach to anemia is necessary and should include a good history, physical examination, and a complete blood count, including blood films. Treatment should be aimed at correcting the primary disorder and supporting the patient. Therefore it is important to establish whether the anemia is *regenerative* or *nonregenerative*. This can be done by obtaining the reticulocyte count. Regenerative anemias are usually the result of hemorrhage or hemolysis, whereas nonregenerative cases may involve the bone marrow.

ANEMIA CAUSED BY HEMORRHAGE

The most common cause of hemorrhage is trauma, although platelet abnormalities and abnormal clotting chemistries must be included. Acute hemorrhage occurring as a result of trauma or laceration is usually an easily diagnosed problem. With acute blood loss the hematocrit does not reflect the severity of the problem, and as fluid shifts occur to compensate for blood loss, shock may result. Treatment should consist of controlling the hemorrhage and volume replacement.

Thrombocytopenia accounts for many cases of generalized bleeding in pet animals. In these cases, it may be more difficult for the veterinarian to diagnose blood loss. Signs of platelet deficiency include petechial hemorrhages on earflaps, mucous membranes, and on nonhaired areas such as the abdomen. Treatment involves steroid therapy, platelet-rich or whole blood transfusions, and avoiding trauma.

IRON-DEFICIENCY ANEMIA

Dogs undergoing chronic external blood loss can develop iron-deficiency anemia. Severe flea infestation, gastrointestinal parasites, gastric ulceration, and bleeding neoplasms can result in significant blood loss over time. The iron and hemoglobin lost with this external bleeding result in the formation of altered red blood cells with decreased life spans. Treatment consists of correcting the cause of the blood loss and supplementing iron orally for 30 to 60 days.

HEMOLYSIS

When immune components attach directly or indirectly to the red cell membrane, they alter its structure. The body, in an attempt to regain homeostasis, begins to remove these altered cells. Macrophages interact with the altered cells, resulting in extravascular hemolysis. This disease, when seen in the dog, seems to be related to the presence of an underlying inflammatory process. Affected animals acutely develop exercise intolerance, pale mucous membranes, tachycardia, and icterus if the condition is severe. In cats, the most common cause of hemolytic anemia is haemobartonellosis. Chronic infections with feline leukemia virus (FeLV) may also stimulate immunohemolytic disease in the cat.

Treatment is aimed at suppressing the immune system (steroid therapy) and supportive therapy. Transfusion should be considered if the hematocrit of the cat falls to life-threatening levels. Tetracycline should be used to treat cats with haemobartonellosis.

A special form of immune-mediated hemolytic disease is seen in neonates. This occurs in horses and, rarely, in cats and dogs. The dam passes antibodies against fetal red blood cells in her colostrum. The neonate's red blood cells are attacked and lysed because they are coated with these antibodies. This problem can be avoided by blood typing breeding animals and by fostering young born to incompatible females.

BLOOD-BORNE PARASITES

Several commonly seen blood parasitic diseases produce anemia through hemolysis. *Haemobartonella felis* is a common cause of anemia in cats. The parasite attaches to the erythrocyte membrane, resulting in increased destruction of the cells. Animals presented with nonspecific signs of weight loss, anorexia, fever, hepatomegaly, and splenomegaly should have blood films examined for the presence of this microorganism. Some of these animals may be icteric on presentation.

Babesia canis and *Babesia gibsoni* both produce hemolytic disease in the dog (Fig. 6-1). The brown dog tick *Rhipicephalus sanguineus* transmits these parasites. The presence of this intracellular parasite results in hemolysis of the infected red cells. Diagnosis is accomplished by finding the intracellular organism on blood films or by serology testing. Symptoms seen in the dog

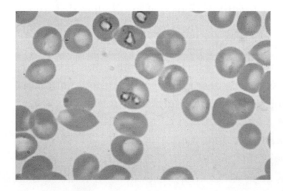

FIGURE 6-1.   Trophozoites of *Babesia canis* within canine red blood cells. (From Hendrix CM: *Diagnostic veterinary parasitology,* ed 2, St Louis, 1998, Mosby.)

include hemoglobinuria, dehydration, fever, anorexia, and depression. Treatment involves tetracycline administration (for haemobartonellosis) and supportive care.

Cytauxzoon felis is a protozoal organism from the southern United States (Florida to Texas and Oklahoma) that is responsible for a fatal disease in cats. The intracellular form of the disease produces an anemia whereas the extracellular form proliferates within the macrophages lining the vascular system, resulting in blood stasis and vascular occlusion. Cats die within days of the development of clinical signs.

TOXIN-INDUCED ANEMIAS

Drugs can be the source of anemias in small animals. One of the most common causes of Heinz body anemia in the dog is onion toxicity, primarily from owners treating the dog to table scraps. Clinical signs may appear several days after ingestion and they are usually those of a mild anemia. Acetaminophen toxicity also results in methemoglobinemia and anemia in dogs and cats. Toxic doses are usually the result of the owner medicating the animal. As little as half a tablet can result in clinical signs. Methylene blue, which is a urinary antiseptic used in cats, has long been known to produce Heinz body anemia when given to normal cats.

Specific diseases of clinical significance include immune-mediated hemolytic anemia, immune-mediated thrombocytopenia, ehrlichiosis, and von Willebrand disease.

IMMUNE-MEDIATED HEMOLYTIC ANEMIA (IMHA)

Although the specific etiology of this disease is unknown, the accelerated red cell destruction occurs owing to the presence of antibodies that attach to the red-cell membrane. These cells are then removed by the immune system, resulting in anemia. The antibodies may bind directly to the cell membrane or may attach to a microorganism or drug that has previously been bound to the membrane receptor sites. Adherence of these antibodies activates the complement system, resulting in agglutination and destruction of the red cell.

IMHA is found most commonly in dogs 2 to 8 years of age. There is a breed predisposition in Poodles, Old English Sheepdogs, Irish Setters, and Cocker Spaniels. The disease is four times more prevalent in females than males.

Clinical syndromes seen with IMHA include immune-mediated extravascular hemolysis, intravascular hemolysis, and cryopathic immune-mediated hemolytic anemia.

CLINICAL SIGNS

- Anorexia
- Listlessness, weakness
- Depression
- Tachycardia, tachypnea
- With or without icterus (if intravascular)
- With or without hepatomegaly, splenomegaly (if extravascular)
- Necrosis of distal extremities (cryopathic form)
- Pale mucous membranes

DIAGNOSIS

- Complete blood count (CBC): Leukocytosis; absolute neutrophilia with a left shift; regenerative anemia

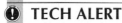

❶ TECH ALERT

Spherocytes are commonly seen on CBC.

- Serum chemistries are usually unremarkable.
- Agglutination test: Mix 1 drop of anticoagulated blood and one drop of saline on a clean glass slide. If antibody molecules are present, agglutination will be observed.
- Direct Coombs test: Must be species specific. False positive and negative results are common. Take clinical signs into account when interpreting a positive result.
- Direct immunofluorescence assay: Detects antibodies against immunoglobulin IgG, IgA, IgM, and complement C3.

TREATMENT

- Treatment should be aimed at improving tissue oxygenation and managing immune response.
- Glucocorticoids: Dexamethasone 1.1 to 0.22 mg/kg IV q 12 h; prednisone or prednisolone 1.1 mg/kg PO q 12 h
- Cimetidine or misoprostol to prevent gastric ulceration from cortisone:
    Cimetidine: 5.5 to 11 mg/kg PO q 6 to 12 h
    Misoprostol: 4.4 to 8.8 g/kg PO q 6 h

- Sucralfate to protect gastric ulcerations: 1g PO q 8 h
- Danazol: A synthetic testosterone that works synergistically with cortisone: 5.5 mg/kg PO q 12 h
- Heparin to prevent thromboembolism or disseminated intravascular coagulation (DIC): 75 µg/kg SQ t.i.d.

INFORMATION FOR CLIENTS
- The prognosis for animals with this disease is guarded.
- Approximately 30% to 40% of all dogs will die despite aggressive treatment.
- Relapses are common.
- Your veterinarian may suggest an ovariohysterectomy for your intact female dog.

IMMUNE-MEDIATED THROMBOCYTOPENIA (IMTP)

As in IMHA, immune-mediated thrombocytopenia occurs when platelets become coated with antibodies or complement-antibody complexes. Destruction may occur in the spleen, bone marrow, or liver. The inciting cause is usually unknown, but some drugs such as sulfonamide, chlorothiazide, arsenicals, digitoxin, and quinidine have been associated with the development of IMTP. The disease typically appears in dogs 5 to 6 years of age; females are 2 times more likely to be affected than males.

As platelet numbers drop below 30,000 thrombocytes/mm^3 of blood, bleeding problems develop. Animals are usually presented for bleeding, most commonly epistaxis. Petechial hemorrhages may appear on mucous membranes, earflaps, and other mucocutaneous surfaces. Bloody stool or blood in vomitus is occasionally seen.

CLINICAL SIGNS
- Petechial and ecchymotic hemorrhages on skin and mucosal surfaces
- Weakness, lethargy

DIAGNOSIS
- Rule out other causes of thrombocytopenia such as DIC, lymphoma, and myeloproliferative disease.
- Bone marrow examination indicates actively budding megakaryocytes and increased plasma cells.
- Clinical signs and response to treatment confirm diagnosis.

TREATMENT

- Prednisone: 2 to 4 mg/kg/day divided b.i.d.
- Vincristine: 0.25 to 0.5 mg/m^2 IV repeated 1 to 2 times at weekly intervals
- Platelet-rich transfusion
- Danazol and cimetidine as for IMHA

INFORMATION FOR CLIENTS

- The prognosis for patients with this disease is guarded to good. About 20% of affected animals will die.
- Relapses may occur.
- Splenectomy may be required in refractory cases.
- Owners of intact females should consider having the pet spayed to decrease hormonal stress.

EHRLICHIOSIS

Ehrlichia canis was first recognized in the United States in 1963. The disease gained prominence owing to the large losses among military working dogs stationed in Vietnam. The disease is seen primarily in tropical and subtropical environments throughout the world.

This rickettsial disease is spread by the tick vector *Rhipicephalus sanguineus*, the brown dog tick, and is most commonly diagnosed in dogs living in the southeastern and southwestern United States, which are areas with large tick populations. Infection occurs when the organism is transmitted via the tick saliva during a blood meal. It may also be transmitted by blood transfusion from an infected to a noninfected patient. After infection the organism multiplies within mononuclear cells, both circulating and fixed (liver, spleen, and lymph nodes). The infected circulating cells can infect other organs. Infection results in vascular endothelial damage, platelet consumption, and erythrocyte destruction. There is also suppression of the bone marrow, resulting in aplastic anemia.

Dogs unable to mount an adequate immune response become chronically infected.

CLINICAL SIGNS

ACUTE PHASE

- Depression, anorexia
- Fever

- Weight loss
- Ocular and nasal discharge
- Dyspnea
- Edema of the limbs or scrotum
- Lymphadenopathy

CHRONIC PHASE
- Bleeding tendencies
- Severe weight loss
- Debilitation
- Abdominal tenderness
- Anterior uveitis, retinal hemorrhages

DIAGNOSIS
HEMATOLOGY
- Pancytopenia
- Aplastic anemia
- Thrombocytopenia (most common sign)
- Anemia
- Positive Coombs test
- Increased serum proteins
- Finding the organisms within peripheral blood smears

SEROLOGY
- IFA test

TREATMENT
- Tetracycline: 22 mg/kg t.i.d. for 14 days is the treatment of choice.
- Doxycycline: 10 mg/kg for 14 days has been used in refractory cases.
- Tetracycline: 6.6 mg/kg daily is used as prophylaxis in endemic areas.

INFORMATION FOR CLIENTS
- The prognosis for this disease is generally good.
- Because dogs do not mount a protective immune response, reinfection may occur.
- Long-term tetracycline prophylaxis may be required in endemic areas.
- Tick control is important to prevent disease.

VON WILLEBRAND DISEASE (vWD)

Canine von Willebrand disease (vWD) is the most common inherited disorder of hemostasis. In normal dogs, von Willebrand factor (vWF) promotes platelet clumping, whereas decreased amounts or lack of the factor results in a bleeding disorder. vWD has been identified in 54 breeds in the United States with Doberman Pinschers, German Shepherds, and Labrador Retrievers being over-represented. In most dogs the inheritance is autosomal dominant with incomplete penetrance. Dogs carrying the gene will demonstrate variable signs and severity with respect to bleeding tendencies.

Dogs with this disorder should not be used for breeding. Special care must be taken at surgery to ensure adequate hemostasis, so it is recommended that breeds that can carry the affected gene have a buccal mucosal bleeding time performed before surgery.

CLINICAL SIGNS
- Easy bruising in breeds predisposed to the disease
- Prolonged bleeding during estrus
- Prolonged bleeding from venipuncture

DIAGNOSIS
- Buccal mucosal bleeding time prolonged >4 minutes
- Low levels of vWF in plasma
- DNA confirmation of the gene defect
- Positive ELISA

TREATMENT
- Bleeding episodes can be managed with plasma or cryoprecipitate infusion.
- Desmopressin acetate can be used to control bleeding during surgery (administer 20 to 30 minutes before surgery). Effect lasts about 2 hours. Dose: 1 to 4 µg/kg SQ

INFORMATION FOR CLIENTS
- This disease is inherited. You should *not* breed this animal.
- Any trauma or stress may precipitate a bleeding episode.
- Surgery will require special precautions to control hemorrhage.
- When purchasing one of the affected breeds, always purchase dogs whose parents have been found to be free of the disease.

LYMPHOMA

FELINE

Lymphoma accounts for approximately 90% of all feline hematopoietic tumors. Most feline lymphomas are induced by FeLV, with 70% of lymphoma cases being FeLV-positive cats. The average age for development of the disease in FeLV-positive cats is 3 years of age, whereas in FeLV-negative cats the disease develops later in life (7 years of age). Cats with the multicentric form of the disease have the greatest incidence of FeLV-positive status (80%).

Lymphomas may be classified in two ways: by anatomic location or according to the extent of the disease. Both schemes complement each other. This chapter concentrates on the classification system using anatomic location.

MEDIASTINAL LYMPHOMA

The mediastinal, or thymic, form is seen in young cats (2 to 3 years of age). Most of these cats are FeLV positive (80%). Clinical signs associated with this form of the disease are those of a space-occupying mass within the mediastinum and include the following: dyspnea, tachypnea, regurgitation, cough, anorexia, depression, weight loss, and pleural effusion.

ALIMENTARY LYMPHOMA

The alimentary form occurs in older cats and the majority of these cats are FeLV negative (70%). Clinical signs are related to an intestinal mass and include the following: vomiting, diarrhea, weight loss, and intestinal obstruction.

MULTICENTRIC LYMPHOMA

Multicentric disease is the most commonly observed form of lymphoma. Most of these cats are FeLV positive, with the average age of presentation being 4 years. Clinical signs are variable and depend on the location and the size of the tumors. Many cats may be asymptomatic, whereas others may have anorexia, weight loss, and lethargy. Peripheral lymph nodes may become visibly enlarged but are nonpainful on palpation. Because a majority of these cats are also FeLV positive, anemia is also prevalent.

CLINICAL SIGNS

Clinical signs depend on the location and size of the tumors but can include the following:

- Dyspnea
- Anemia
- Vomiting
- Diarrhea
- Lethargy
- Weight loss
- Visibly enlarged peripheral lymph nodes

DIAGNOSIS

- Cytology is the best method for diagnosis. Fine needle aspirates or surgical biopsy will provide a diagnosis. Cytology will reveal a monomorphic population of immature lymphocytes.

TREATMENT

- Chemotherapy is the preferred method of treatment. Drug protocols are divided into four phases: induction of remission, intensification, maintenance, and rescue.

INDUCTION OF REMISSION

- COP (Cytoxan, Oncovin, prednisone) protocol:
    Cyclophosphamide (Cytoxan): 300 mg/m^2 PO given on days 1 and 22 of the month
    Vincristine (Oncovin): 0.75 mg/m^2 IV given on days 1, 8, 15, and 22 of the month
    Prednisone: 2 mg/kg once daily

❶ TECH ALERT

Remission rates of up to 80% have been reported with this protocol; the duration of remission ranges from 42 days to 42 months.

- COAP (Cytoxan, Oncovin, cytosine arabinoside, prednisone) protocol:
    Cyclophosphamide (Cytoxan): 50 mg/m^2 PO 4 days/week given every other day
    Vincristine (Oncovin): 0.5 mg/m^2 IV once each week
    Cytosine arabinoside (Cytostar-U): 100 mg/m^2/day given by IV drip or SQ for only 2 days

Prednisone: 40 mg/m^2 PO daily for 7 days then 20 mg/m^2 every other day

Use protocol for 6 weeks, then switch to maintenance therapy.

INTENSIFICATION

- Add L-asparaginase (Elspar) 10,000 to 20,000 IU/m^2 SQ for one dose.

MAINTENANCE

- LMP (Leukeran, methotrexate, prednisone) protocol:

    Chlorambucil (Leukeran): 2 mg/m^2 PO every other day or 20 mg/m^2 PO every other week

    Methotrexate: 2.5 mg/m^2 PO, 2 to 3 times weekly

    Prednisone: 20 mg/m^2 PO every other day

RESCUE

- Protocols are available that add drugs such as adriamycin and dacarbazine (see the literature).

Additional drugs used in the treatment of lymphomas in the cat include the following:

- Idarubicin: 2 mg/day for 2 consecutive days every 21 days
- Doxorubicin: 25 mg/m^2 IV every 3 weeks

RADIATION THERAPY

- Useful in cases of localized lymphomas

❶ TECH ALERT

Note that doses are in mg/m^2. Body surface area is a more accurate method of dosing toxic materials.

- All the chemotherapeutic agents induce side effects in animals undergoing treatment. These include the following:

    Anorexia: Use cyproheptadine 4 to 8 mg b.i.d. to t.i.d. to stimulate appetite.

    Vomiting

    Leukopenia: Check blood count 1 week after each dose of Cytoxan. Reduce the dose by 25% if segmented neutrophil count is <1000 cells/μl.

    Renal toxicity: Monitor renal function.

    Hemorrhagic cystitis: This is uncommon but can occur with Cytoxan.

INFORMATION FOR CLIENTS

- There is *no* cure for this disease. The goal of therapy is to induce remission, make the cat more comfortable, and prolong life.
- Cats that achieve complete remission live a median of 5 months (with a range of 2 to 42 months); all animals will have a relapse of the disease eventually.
- Maintenance therapy and follow-up is important to the success of the treatment protocol.
- Nutritional support is important with the alimentary form of the disease; a feeding tube may be needed.
- All therapy protocols will produce some toxicity that may need to be treated.
- Wear gloves when handling chemotherapeutic drugs to prevent absorption through the skin.

⊕ TECH ALERT

Clinicians and technicians should consult with oncology specialists for optional protocols in the treatment of this disease.

CANINE

Malignant lymphoma (lymphosarcoma) is the most common hematopoietic tumor of the dog. More than 85% of cases seen by veterinarians involve regional or generalized lymphadenopathy. Survival times for untreated dogs are short and most die within 4 to 6 weeks after diagnosis. With treatment, remission rates can approach 90%; the duration of remission normally lasts longer than 6 months.

Therapy involves two phases of treatment: the induction and maintenance phase and the rescue phase. Combined drug protocols provide the best response rates and duration of remission. Dogs treated initially with only prednisolone have shorter remission periods and decreased survival times. The reader is referred to the literature for the various protocols available. Eventually most dogs will require rescue therapy.

The duration of the new remissions is generally poor owing to the emergence of drug-resistant tumor cells.

Alternative therapies such as monoclonal antibody therapy or bone marrow transplants show some promise for future treatment of this disease in the dog.

CLINICAL SIGNS

- Enlarged peripheral lymph nodes
- Lethargy
- Weight loss
- Vomiting and/or diarrhea

DIAGNOSIS

- Cytology/biopsy (similar to the cat)

TREATMENT

- Several combined drug therapy protocols are available. The one listed here is from the University of Wisconsin at Madison:

  Vincristine: 0.7 mg/m^2 IV weeks 1, 3, 6, and 8

  L-Asparaginase: 400 IU/kg IM week 1

  Prednisone: PO daily weeks 1, 2, 3, and 4

  (2 mg/kg/day, week 1; 1.5 mg/kg/day, week 2; 1 mg/kg/day, week 3; 0.5 mg/kg/day, week 4)

  Cyclophosphamide (Cytoxan): 200 mg/m^2 IV weeks 2 and 7

  Doxorubicin: 30 mg/m^2 IV weeks 4 and 9

Other treatments that may result in less successful remissions include the following:

- Prednisone: 1 to 2 mg/kg/day PO; this treatment has been shown to help for a short period of time (30 days), but use of it may make it more difficult to reestablish remission a second time.
- Cytoxan: 50 mg/m^2 PO for 4 consecutive days weekly. Give with prednisone.
- Doxorubicin: 30 mg/m^2 IV every 3 weeks for a total of five treatments.

MAINTENANCE THERAPY

- Vincristine: 0.7 mg/m^2 IV
- Chlorambucil: 1.4 mg/kg PO
- Methotrexate 0.8 mg/kg IV or doxorubicin 30 mg/m^2 IV (alternate these two drugs until a total doxorubicin dose of 180 mg/m^2 is attained, then use methotrexate alone):

  Begin on week 11 and alternate these three treatments every 2 weeks.

  After week 25, alternate every 3 weeks.

  After week 49, alternate every 4 weeks.

  Discontinue after 2 years if the dog is in complete remission.

RESCUE THERAPY
- Actinomycin D: 0.9 to 1.1 mg/m^2 IV every 2 to 3 weeks
- Mitoxantrone: 5 to 6 mg/m^2 every 3 weeks
- Doxorubicin (30 mg/m^2 IV day 1) and dacarbazine (200 mg/m^2 IV days 1 to 5). Cycle every 21 days.

INFORMATION FOR CLIENTS
- Most dogs will eventually relapse.
- Durability of new remissions is usually poor; life expectancy ranges from 2 to 5 months.
- Medications used in chemotherapy will cause suppression of the immune system and blood counts will need to be monitored frequently.
- Boxers, Bull Mastiffs, Basset Hounds, Saint Bernards, and Scottish Terriers have a predisposition for this disease.
- Without treatment, most dogs die within 4 to 6 weeks following diagnosis.
- With proper treatment, survival time may approach 1 year.

FELINE IMMUNODEFICIENCY VIRUS (FIV, FELINE AIDS)

Feline immunodeficiency virus (FIV) was first isolated in 1987 by Pederson and colleagues. The virus, a lentivirus, interacts with lymphocytes (predominantly CD4+ cells and macrophages), changing their ability to function normally in the immune response process. The resulting lymphopenia, loss of memory cell function, and decrease in antibody production from T-cell stimulated lymphocytes leaves the cat open for opportunistic infections.

FIV is endemic in most of the United States. Outdoor, free-roaming cats are most at risk, with males being 1.5 to 3 times more likely to become infected than females. This is probably related to their fighting behavior and territorial aggressiveness. The average age at the time of diagnosis is between 6 and 8 years. Incidental transmission through food bowls, mutual grooming, or other fomites is unlikely in multiple cat households. Kittens can become infected with the virus while nursing queens that are experiencing the acute phase of the disease (FIV passed in milk).

The disease can be divided into three stages: acute infection (3 to 6 months), subclinical infection (months to years), and chronic clinical infection (months to years).
- **Acute stage:** Usually mild symptoms of recurrent fever, lethargy, anorexia, and generalized lymphadenopathy.

- **Subclinical stage:** Usually no clinical signs shown in infected cats. However, the disease is progressing.
- **Chronic clinical stage:** A variety of signs involve the establishment of opportunistic infections throughout the body and symptoms related to viral infection:
    Chronic stomatitis and weight loss
    Recurrent upper respiratory tract infections
    Chronic enteritis
    Persistent dermatomycosis
    Ocular disease—anterior uveitis, retinal degeneration/hemorrhage, transient conjunctivitis
    Tumors
    Chronic wasting syndrome—cats lose up to 30% of body weight in several weeks
    Neurologic signs—altered behavior, paresis, weakness

Therapies are focused on preventing exposure to pathogens and supportive care. The average time from diagnosis to death is approximately 5 years.

CLINICAL SIGNS
- Febrile episodes
- Lymphadenopathy
- Persistent infections unresponsive to treatment
- Weight loss
- Gingivitis
- Ocular lesions
- Slow-healing traumatic wounds
- Behavior abnormalities
- Chronic upper respiratory infections
- Anemia

DIAGNOSIS
- In-house serology: Membrane-bound ELISA test (CITE test, Idexx) is sensitive and specific for the presence of antibodies.

TREATMENT
- Reverse transcriptase inhibitors—expensive and easily available:
    Azothiouridine (AZT, Retrovir, Burroughs Wellcome): 10 mg/ kg t.i.d.

Interferon-α: 0.5 to 30 U/cat PO q 24 h for 5 days on alternate weeks

SUPPORTIVE CARE
- Limit contact with other cats to decrease exposure to secondary pathogens.
- Avoid routine vaccinations.
- Limit vaccines to rabies as required by law.

PREVENTIVE
- Keep cats inside; avoid contact with feral cats.

INFORMATION FOR CLIENTS
- This is a progressive disease.
- The average life span from diagnosis to death is about 5 years.
- To prevent this disease, keep cats indoors and limit contact with feral or free-roaming cats.
- Test all new additions to the cat's household.
- Incidental infection among cats in a household is unlikely.
- FIV has not been found to grow in human cells.

Diseases of the Integumentary System

The skin makes up the largest organ system in the body. It comprises approximately 24% of the total body weight of a newborn puppy and about 12% of the body weight of an adult animal. It consists of three distinct layers—the *epidermis,* the *dermis*, and the *hypodermis,* or subcuticular layer (Fig. 7-1). (The technician should refer to an anatomy and physiology textbook for the exact function of each layer.) The skin serves as a barrier between the animal's body and the environment. It not only protects the animal from physical, chemical, and microbiological injury, but the sensory organs found in the skin allow the animal to feel pain, heat, cold, touch, and pressure. The skin is also a storage depot for electrolytes, water, proteins, fats, and carbohydrates, and it assists in the activation of vitamin D by solar energy.

The hypodermis stores fat for insulation and energy reserves. The animal's skin has many functions:

- *Enclosing barrier:* Protects the internal environment of the body from water and electrolyte loss.
- *Environmental protection:* Protects the internal environment from the external environment.
- *Temperature regulation:* Maintains the animal's coat and regulates the blood supply to the cutaneous tissues, which regulates heat dissipation and retention.
- *Sensory perception:* Contains sense organs for touch, temperature, and pain.
- *Motion and shape:* Allows for motion and provides a definition to the body.
- *Antimicrobial:* Contains antimicrobial and antifungal properties.
- *Blood pressure control:* The peripheral vascular beds within the skin help control blood pressure.
- *Secretion:* Contains both apocrine and sebaceous glands.
- *Adnexa:* Produces hair, nails, hooves, and horny layers of the epidermis.

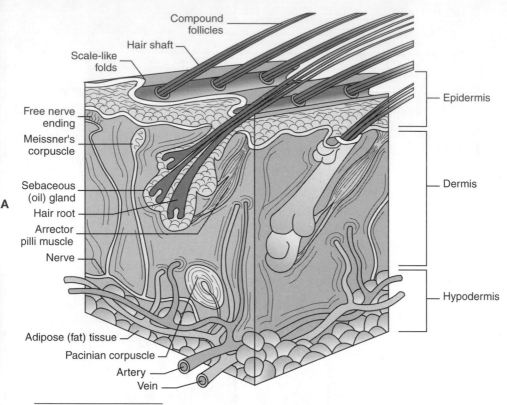

FIGURE 7-1.   A, Canine skin and underlying subcutaneous tissue. Notice that epidermis of canine skin includes folds from which compound hairs arise. (**A,** From Colville T, Bassert JM: *Clinical anatomy and physiology for veterinary technicians,* St Louis, 2002, Mosby.)

- *Storage:* Stores electrolytes, water, vitamins, fat, proteins, carbohydrates, and other substances.
- *Pigmentation:* Processes within the skin (e.g., melanin formation) help determine coat and skin color and provide solar protection.
- *Excretion:* Has a limited excretory function.
- *Vitamin D production:* Essential for solar energy activation of vitamin D, which is necessary for normal calcium absorption.

🛈 TECH ALERT
The skin is an important indicator of internal disease.

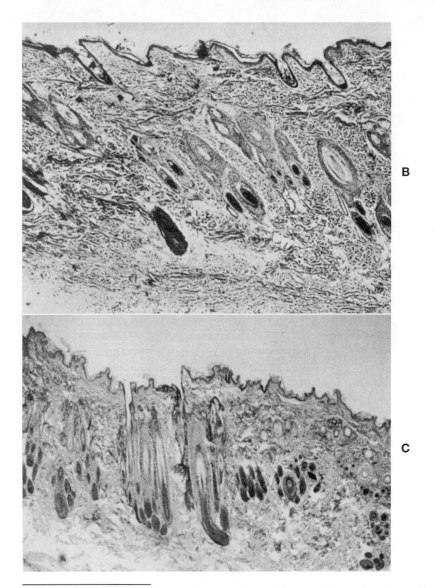

FIGURE 7-1, CONT'D. **B,** Normal canine skin. **C,** Normal feline skin. Note the thin epidermis and compound hair follicle arrangement of both species. (**B** and **C,** from Scott DW, Miller WH, Jr., Griffin CE: *Muller and Kirk's small animal dermatology,* ed 6, Philadelphia, 2001, WB Saunders.)

Any physical condition that disrupts the normal functions of this barrier can result in disease. Increased moisture, chemical exposure, increased temperature, hormonal change, and physical damage can produce a breach in the barrier, allowing the invasion of disease-producing microorganisms.

Problems relating to the skin are the most frequent complaints presented in small animal medicine. Technicians deal with these complaints daily as clients ask questions and seek help for the treatment and prevention of skin diseases afflicting their pets. This chapter will focus on the most commonly seen skin problems of companion animals.

ECTOPARASITES

External parasites are responsible for many skin problems seen in small animal medicine. The technician is referred to a parasitology text for detailed information on the life cycles of the individual parasites discussed in this chapter. The most commonly diagnosed ectoparasites are as follows:

- Ear mites   (*Otodectes cynotis*)
- Fleas   (*Ctenocephalides* spp.)
- Ticks   (*Ixodes* spp., and others)
- Mange   (*Demodex canis, Sarcoptes scabiei, Notoedres cati*)
- Warbles   (*Cutebrae* spp.)
- Myiasis   (fly maggots)
- Lice   (*Linognathus setosus*)

Some of these parasites live on the skin, some live within or under the skin, and some pierce the skin, sucking blood meals that produce severe cutaneous reactions. These reactions include inflammation, edema, and itching. In many cases, the animal itself is responsible for increased damage to the skin through licking, chewing, and scratching.

EAR MITES *(OTODECTES CYNOTIS)*

These mites live on the surface of the skin in the external ear canal, feeding on epidermal debris (Fig. 7-2).

CLINICAL SIGNS
- Ear canals may be filled with a brown-black, crusty exudate.
- Mites are extremely irritating, so animals will scratch their ears.
- Scrapes (wounds) may be visible on the side of the face or head.

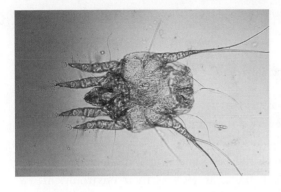

FIGURE 7-2.   Adult male ear mite, *Otodectes cynotis*. (From Hendrix CM: *Diagnostic veterinary parasitology*, ed 2, St Louis, 1998, Mosby.)

DIAGNOSIS
- Under an otoscope, the large, white, adult mites can be seen crawling on the surface of the crusty exudate.
- Adult mites and eggs can be seen on microscopic examination of smears taken of the exudate.

TREATMENT
- Many otic products contain ingredients that will kill mites. The technician should first carefully clean the exudate from the ear canal, then apply a miticide into the canal. Recommended miticides include the following:

    Tresaderm: 5 to 15 drops b.i.d. topically to ear canals

    Mitox: Fill lower canal once daily; massage to distribute medication

    Otomite: 4 to 15 drops daily in ear canals

    Ivermectin (off-label use): 300 µg/kg SQ or PO *(repeat in 14 days)*

❶ TECH ALERT
Owners must be informed that ivermectin is not licensed for subcutaneous use in companion animal species.

INFORMATION FOR CLIENTS
- The life cycle of the parasite is 3 weeks. Eggs hatch every 10 days, so treatment must be continued for no less than 30 days.
- This parasite is highly contagious. All animals having contact with the infested animal should be treated.
- Humans do not become infested with this parasite in most cases.
- The mites may spend time elsewhere on the animal's body—especially

on a cat's tail. If infestations recur, treat the entire animal with dip or shampoo.

FLEAS (*CTENOCEPHALIDES* SPP.)

Fleas are blood-sucking ectoparasites that feed sporadically on mammals and birds (Fig. 7-3). Fleas produce severe skin irritation as a result of their frequent bites. Flea saliva is highly antigenic in some animals and will produce an allergic dermatitis. Fleas can act as vectors for diseases and as intermediary hosts for the dog tapeworm *(Dipylidium canium)*. Pets, as well as their environment, can become infested with massive numbers of fleas.

CLINICAL SIGNS
- Animals infested with fleas will continually scratch or bite at their skin.
- Areas commonly affected include the tail-head area and the inner thigh region of the animal. These areas may be red, inflamed, and scabbed. In cats, small scabs may cover the entire dorsum (miliary dermatitis).
- Small, pepperlike granules may be found on the skin and hair coat. When placed on white paper wet with alcohol or water, the granules give off a red color. These granules are dried flea excrement, which contain blood products.

DIAGNOSIS
- Finding fleas on the animal
- Finding flea dirt on the animal
- Finding lesions consistent with flea infestation

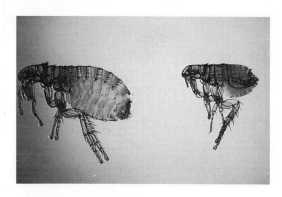

FIGURE 7-3. Adult male and female *Ctenocephalides felis,* cat fleas, the most common flea found on dogs and cats. (From Hendrix CM: *Diagnostic veterinary parasitology,* ed 2, St Louis, 1998, Mosby.)

TREATMENT

- Several flea products are on the market. They can be broken down into those that are applied topically (sprays, dips, powders, and shampoos) and those that are applied systemically (spot-ons, oral, or injectable). All these products act at some point in the flea's life cycle to interrupt development of the adult flea or to repel the adult flea from the animal.

SPRAYS AND POWDERS

- Many products containing a combination of ingredients are on the market. Most act to repel or kill the adult flea. Each product has specific species and age specifications, so read the label carefully before use. Become familiar with the products sold in your clinic.

SHAMPOOS

- Shampoos provide no residual effect. The product will kill fleas that come into contact with the shampoo, but it will not remain on the skin after rinsing. Read the label carefully for species specifications.

DIPS

- Dips provide residual effect on the animal. These products are more toxic than other topical preparations. Read the label carefully for species specifications and proper dilution techniques.

SYSTEMICS

- Systemics are one of the newest treatments for fleas. These products are absorbed and distributed within the skin to kill the flea when it feeds, or it renders reproduction impossible.

  Advantage: A once monthly spot-on that kills adult fleas and prevents reproduction. Dosed according to weight and species.

  Program: Lufenuron, the active ingredient, is absorbed by the fatty tissue and slowly distributed to the bloodstream. This ingredient interferes with the synthesis of chitin, a necessary element in flea development. Given by tablet once monthly or every 6 months by injection to cats. Takes 30 to 60 days to reach full effectiveness. Adult fleas may continue to be seen on the animal.

  Frontline: Apply monthly to skin.

  Sentinel: Contains lufenuron. Also contains milbemycin for heartworm prevention. Dosed by weight in dogs.

Revolution (selamectin, Pfizer): Kills fleas for 1 month by preventing the eggs from hatching. It is also used to treat heartworms, ear mites, intestinal parasites, and sarcoptic mange in dogs and cats >6 weeks of age. Dosed by body weight.

INFORMATION FOR CLIENTS

- Control of ectoparasites such as fleas can be a frustrating task. Environmental factors, geographic location, and species sensitivity affect the development of disease.
- Treatment of the environment is essential in preventing flea infestation. Fleas spend most of their life cycle off the host.
- If one animal in the house has fleas, they all have fleas!
- Flea infestation results in damage to the skin, allowing other skin problems to develop.
- Fleas will bite and feed on humans if animals are not available.
- Some fleas can remain dormant in the environment for months if conditions are right. You must clean the environment by vacuuming and treating with sprays or foggers.

TICKS (*IXODES* SPP. AND *ARGASID* SPP.)

Ticks are seen commonly on outdoor dogs and cats, especially during the summer months. These blood-sucking, arthropod parasites are not host specific and will infest all warm-blooded animals in the area (including humans). Heavy infestation may produce anemia in the host. Ticks also can transmit many bacterial, viral, rickettsial, and protozoan diseases. Lyme disease is one high profile example of tick-borne disease. Ticks are divided into two main families: Ixodidae (hard ticks) and Argasidae (soft ticks). Most of the commonly found ticks belong to the Ixodidae family. Some of the best known members of this family include *Rhipicephalus sanguineus* (the brown dog tick [Fig. 7-4]), *Dermacentor variabilis* (the American dog tick), and *Amblyomma* spp. All but *Rhipicephalus* spp. gain access to the host outdoors. *Rhipicephalus* spp. typically inhabit buildings and kennels. One soft tick, the spinose ear tick *(Otobius megnini)* can be found in the ear canals of dogs and cats in the southwestern United States.

Ticks injure animals by several means: irritation of the actual bite, as vectors of disease, and through a neurotoxin found in the saliva of twelve different *Ixodes* species. This neurotoxin causes *tick paralysis,* an ascending, flaccid paralysis of dogs.

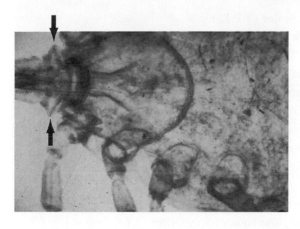

Figure 7-4. *Rhipicephalus sanguineus* (brown dog tick) invades both kennel and household environments. (From Hendrix CM: *Diagnostic veterinary parasitology,* ed 2, St Louis, 1998, Mosby.)

CLINICAL SIGNS

- Owners report a tick or "a lump" attached to the animal
- Weakness or pale mucous membranes when infested with large numbers of ticks
- Ascending, flaccid paralysis
- Arthritis-like symptoms of lameness, joint and muscle pain, fever (Lyme disease)

DIAGNOSIS

- Finding a tick on the animal is the definitive diagnosis.
- A history of exposure to wooded, grassy areas known to have tick infestations suggests the diagnosis.

TREATMENT

- Manual removal of all ticks. Soak the tick in alcohol; firmly grasp the head parts using a curved mosquito hemostat and pull to remove the tick. Destroy the tick by crushing or soaking in alcohol. One should never use bare hands to remove a tick or crush a tick because the blood contained within the tick may contain infectious microorganisms. *Never* use a lighted cigarette, gasoline, or kerosene to remove a tick, as their use will result in serious damage to the skin.
- Topical treatments (dips, sprays, and powders): The list given is only an example of some of the more commonly used products:
  Paramite Dip (Vet-Kem)
  Pyrethrin Dip (VetMate)
  Durakyl Pet Dip (D.V.M.)
  Adams Flea and Tick Dust

       VIP Flea and Tick Powder (V.P.L.)

       Adams Flea and Tick 14-day Mist

- Collars: Preventic collar (Virbac, Inc.) is the only collar that is effective against ticks (even though others claim to be). These collars are effective for about 3 months if they do not get wet.
- Topical systemic treatments: Frontline is a spot-on product effective against fleas.
- Environmental treatments include the following:

       Adams Home and Kennel Spray

       Vet-Fog Fogger

       Siphotrol Plus Fogger

       Permectrin Pet, Yard, and Kennel Spray (Bio-Ceutic)

       Some yard sprays and garden sprays will also kill ticks

- By removing brush, limiting rodent populations, and keeping grassy areas cut, you can decrease the tick population in the environment.

INFORMATION FOR CLIENTS

- Routinely check all animals for ticks, especially after they spend time outside during the spring and summer. Check around the ears and between the toes, as these are areas where ticks are commonly found.
- Do *not* use gasoline, kerosene, or lighted cigarettes to remove ticks from the animal.
- Do *not* use your bare hands to remove or to crush ticks.
- You will need to treat the environment to prevent reinfestation of your pets.
- If infestation is severe, you may need to call a professional exterminator.
- Ticks are not species specific; they will feed on humans whenever they get the chance. They can carry disease.
- Destroy outdoor habitat by cutting brush, trimming trees, and eliminating rodents. Repellant collars and sprays may help keep ticks off pets while outdoors.

MANGE

Three primary diseases called "mange" are seen in the dog and cat: demodectic mange, sarcoptic mange, and notoedric mange. These diseases are the result of tiny mites living on or in the skin where they produce irritation and inflammation. The symptoms for each of the diseases are distinct, and diagnosis must include identification of the mite through skin scrapings or biopsy.

DEMODECTIC MANGE

This cigar-shaped mite, *Demodex canis*, lives within the hair follicles of most dogs and some cats (Fig. 7-5). The mites spend their entire life cycle on the host. In most dogs, the immune system holds the number of mites in check; however, in dogs with compromised immune systems (such as puppies with poor nutrition or other parasites, or dogs with chronic disease) the number of mites becomes excessive, resulting in disease. There seems to be a hereditary predisposition to this disease, and certain breeds seem to be more affected.

Demodectic mange occurs in two forms: *localized*, the more commonly seen form, and *generalized,* the more severe but less common form.

CLINICAL SIGNS (LOCALIZED *DEMODEX*)

- Patient is almost always a young dog (3 months to 1 year). When found in the localized form in adults, the animals have a history of the disease earlier in life.
- Alopecia (hair loss)—especially on the face, around the eyes, mouth, and ears. The next most frequently involved areas are the forelegs and, occasionally, the trunk.
- Erythema (redness)—the patches are red and sometimes crusty. This type of mange has been called *red mange*.

❶ TECH ALERT

The animals are *nonpruritic* (not itching). This is an important distinguishing characteristic to help differentiate demodectic mange from other types.

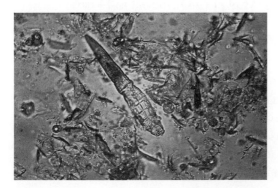

FIGURE 7-5.   Adult *Demodex canis.* These mites resemble eight-legged alligators. (From Hendrix CM: *Diagnostic veterinary parasitology,* ed 2, St Louis, 1998, Mosby.)

CLINICAL SIGNS (GENERALIZED *DEMODEX*)
- Animals will usually be febrile.
- The entire body surface will be involved.
- Secondary bacterial skin infections with pustules will be seen.

DIAGNOSIS
- Diagnosis is by mite identification, usually through skin scrapings. Place a drop of mineral oil on the lesion and firmly scrape while squeezing the skin. Transfer the material to a clean glass slide and examine under a microscope. This mite is easily found.
- Culture and sensitivity of the skin lesions may be necessary if a secondary bacterial infection is present.

TREATMENT
- Treatment of *Demodex* depends on the age of the patient, the extent of the lesions, and veterinarian preference.

LOCALIZED
- Goodwinol ointment: Apply to lesions daily
- Canex: Apply to lesions daily

GENERALIZED OR SEVERE LOCALIZED
- Mitaban dips (Amitraz): Clip the dog closely to remove hair. Bathe the entire animal in a mild soap and towel dry. Treat the entire animal with the dip at the proper dilution (1 bottle/2 gal of water). Do not rinse or towel dry the animal. Three to six treatments may be required, each treatment given 14 days apart and continued until skin scrapings are negative.
- Ivermectin: *Use of this drug in the dog is "off-label," and client release forms should be signed.* Give 0.3 mg/kg SQ or PO. Repeat in 14 days.
- Interceptor: 0.5 to 1.0 mg/kg monthly for a minimum of 90 days
- Oral antibiotics: Choice based on culture and sensitivity

INFORMATION FOR CLIENTS
- Many animals will outgrow mange as they age.
- *Demodex* is not contagious to humans and other animals.
- Treatment will never completely remove the mites from the skin. The goal of treatment is to reduce the number of mites on the animal and to improve the general health of the pet.

- Breeders should not use previously infected animals in their breeding programs.
- Treatment may be prolonged in some animals.
- The generalized form may be fatal in some animals.

SARCOPTIC MANGE (SCABIES)

Scabies is an intensely pruritic, contagious disease of animals. The mite, *Sarcoptes scabiei var. canis,* has a rounded body with four pairs of legs (Fig. 7-6). The female mite burrows into the epidermis, laying eggs. This burrowing produces intense itching and inflammation within the skin. Scabies can occur in dogs of any age, sex, or breed. Humans may develop visible lesions after exposure to infected animals; however, the mites do not survive off the animal host for longer than a few days. If the owner develops small, red papules on his or her skin, a medical doctor should be consulted.

CLINICAL SIGNS
- Typical red, crusty lesions appear on the ears, elbows, and elsewhere on the trunk of the animal.
- *Intensely pruritic!* This distinguishes it from *Demodex*.
- Secondary bacterial skin infections may be present owing to self-trauma.
- The disease will progressively become more severe.

DIAGNOSIS
- Identification of the mite through skin scrapings. These mites are difficult to find in many cases because they are located deep in the epidermis. Scraping should be deep to maximize the chance of finding the mite.

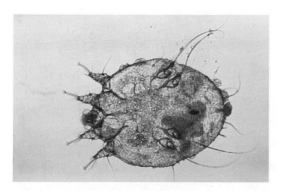

FIGURE 7-6. Adult *Sarcoptes scabiei* mite that causes scabies, an intensely pruritic disease. (From Hendrix CM: *Diagnostic veterinary parasitology,* ed 2, St Louis, 1998, Mosby.)

Multiple scrapings of the same animal may be necessary to locate the mite. Mites can also be seen on skin biopsies.

TREATMENT

- Remove the mites! Dips are frequently used for this purpose.

    Paramite Dip (Vet-Kem): Dip every 14 days until the clinical signs resolve.

    Ivermectin: 0.3 mg/kg SQ or PO. Repeat in 14 days. *This constitutes "off-label" use of this drug.*

    Paramite Dust: Administer per package instructions. Rub through entire coat. Do not treat puppies less than 12 weeks of age.

INFORMATION FOR CLIENTS

- This is a highly contagious disease among dogs.
- Humans frequently develop visible lesions appearing as small, red papules. Owners should contact their doctor if this occurs.
- Mites do not remain on the human for longer than a few hours.
- A similar disease is seen in cats, but the mite is not the same. *Notoedres cati* produces lesions in cats similar to those seen with sarcoptic mange in dogs. The dog mite will rarely infect the cat.
- Species variants of the sarcoptic mite infest almost all species of haired animals.

CUTEREBRA "WARBLES"

The *Cuterebra* fly lays eggs in the soil. These eggs mature into a larval stage similar to a grub that directly penetrates the host's skin (Fig. 7-7). Here, in a subcutaneous pocket, the larva continues to mature, finally leaving the wound to become an adult fly. A fistula or opening in the swelling allows the larva to breathe while maturing; the larva can be seen moving up and down in the opening to the fistula.

DIAGNOSIS

- This disease is usually seen in young puppies, kittens, and rabbits.
- Owners may notice a large swelling behind the ears, on the neck, or around the face. In rabbits, the lesion may be in the nasal cavity.
- The swelling has an opening (a fistula) through which the larva can be seen.

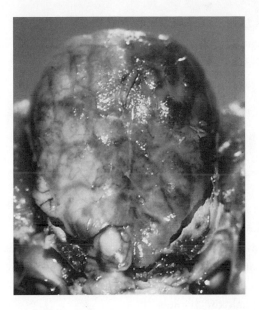

Figure 7-7. *Cuterebra* species, "warbles" or "wolves," found in skin of dogs or cats. (From Hendrix CM: *Diagnostic veterinary parasitology,* ed 2, St Louis, 1998, Mosby.)

TREATMENT
- The fistula opening should be incised to allow removal of the larva. Using a curved mosquito hemostat, carefully remove the intact larva. Avoid crushing or tearing the larva as release of larval protein can cause allergic reactions in the host.
- The wound should be flushed; use diluted Betadine or Nolvasan solution.
- Oral or topical antibiotics should be given to combat skin infection.

INFORMATION FOR CLIENTS
- Keep young animals in clean, fly-free areas to avoid infection.
- Fly repellant gels may help prevent the disease. Apply to ears and around the neck area (read label for restrictions).
- Even after removal of the larva, the wound may heal slowly.

MYIASIS (MAGGOTS)

Many adult forms of dipterous flies often deposit eggs on the wet, warm, or damaged skin of animals. These eggs hatch into larvae known as maggots, which are highly destructive, producing punched-out areas in the skin. These lesions often coalesce to form even larger ulcerated areas. Large numbers of maggots may be found in wounds that have gone unnoticed by owners. Heavy coats and neglect predispose animals to this problem.

DIAGNOSIS
- Owners often report matted hair, a bad odor, or a painful reaction when the animal is petted in a specific area.
- Observing the maggots on physical examination

TREATMENT
- Clip hair from all lesions.
- Flush the areas with copious amounts of water to remove larvae.
- Manually remove larvae not washed off.
- Daily wound cleaning and treatment must be done.
- Administer oral antibiotics to combat the infection; use one with a good spectrum for skin (Keflex, cephalexin, triple sulfas).
- Keep the pet indoors to prevent reinfestation.

INFORMATION FOR CLIENTS
- This is a disease of neglect. Owners need to check their outdoor pets frequently, especially during the summer months.
- Heavy-coated animals should be clipped during the hot, humid summer months to avoid damage to the skin.
- Avoid using toxic dips or sprays on wounds to remove the larvae.
- Keep pets indoors during peak fly hours to prevent infestation (usually early morning and late afternoon).
- Keep pet's outdoor environment clean to avoid attracting flies.

LICE

Lice are host specific and spend all their lives on that host (Fig. 7-8). They are found on debilitated, dirty, ill-kept animals and are commonly seen on poultry and pigeons. This is a disease of neglect.

DIAGNOSIS
- Pet may become ill-tempered, agitated due to the presence of the lice.
- Lice cause intense itching.
- Anemia can develop from blood-sucking lice.
- Presence of lice or nits on the hair coat is diagnostic (Fig. 7-9).

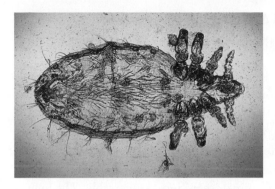

FIGURE 7-8.   Sucking louse *Linognathus setosus* of dogs. (From Hendrix CM: *Diagnostic veterinary parasitology,* ed 2, St Louis, 1998, Mosby.)

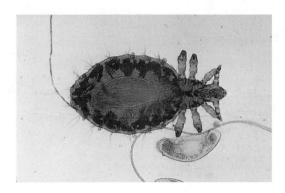

FIGURE 7-9.   *Linognathus setosus;* gravid female sucking louse and associated nit on hair shaft collected from a dog. Nits are oval, white, and usually found cemented to hair shaft. (From Hendrix CM: *Diagnostic veterinary parasitology,* ed 2, St Louis, 1998, Mosby.)

TREATMENT

- Treat all the animals in the house using an insecticide dip, shampoo, or dust. Clip all the hair on the animal. Bathe with a good shampoo. Treat with an insecticide dip, dust, or spray.
- All bedding and grooming tools must be washed thoroughly.
- Ivermectin can be used orally at 0.3 mg/kg. *However, this use is "off-label," so obtain a release from the owner.*

INFORMATION FOR CLIENTS

- Humans cannot get lice from pets.
- The pet cannot get lice from humans.
- Clean the environment to prevent reinfestation.
- Improve the coat care of the pet by including routine bathing and grooming.

SUPERFICIAL DERMATOMYCOSES (FUNGAL INFECTIONS)

Infections by fungal elements usually occur when the dermatophyte penetrates the skin and begins to proliferate on the surface of the hair shaft. Three species of fungi typically cause disease in the dog and cat: *Microsporum gypseum, Trichophyton mentagrophytes,* and *Microsporum canis.* The latter organism is the most commonly isolated dermatophyte of dogs and cats. This fungus may also produce lesions in humans. Infections are usually the result of contact with the organism, and young or debilitated animals seem most susceptible. The fungus produces enzymes that result in hypertrophy of the surrounding epidermis. Lesions become scaly with excessive keratin.

MICROSPORUM CANIS INFECTIONS

CLINICAL SIGNS
- Appearance of a rapidly growing circular patch of alopecia; some areas will be red, raised, and crusty (Fig. 7-10).
- Lesions are most frequently seen on the face and head.
- Hairs in the lesion may appear broken.
- Pet owners may describe similar lesions on themselves.

DIAGNOSIS
- A Wood's light examination may reveal infected hair shafts that fluoresce. Approximately 50% of *M. canis* organisms will be fluorescent on examination. (Hair shaft will glow yellow-green under UV light. Ointments and creams applied topically may also fluoresce, producing a false positive result.)

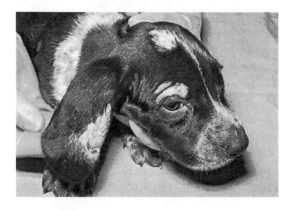

FIGURE 7-10. Pointer puppy with well-circumscribed areas of alopecia and grayish crusts above the eye and on the pinna caused by *Microsporum canis.* (From Scott DW, Miller WH, Jr., Griffin CE: *Muller and Kirk's small animal dermatology,* ed 6, Philadelphia, 2001, WB Saunders.)

- KOH slide preparation: Place hairs and skin scraping on a clean microscope slide and add a few drops of 10% potassium hydroxide. Apply a coverslip and heat gently for a few seconds. Observe for fungal elements.
- Culture: Fungal cultures are the most accurate method of diagnosis. Fungal growth is slow, and it may be 10 to 14 days before results are seen.
- Products such as Fungassay and Sab-Duets (Bacti-labs) may be used in the clinic. A color change from yellow to red occurs with the growth of pathologic organisms. Dermatophyte colonies will be white to cream colored. Cultures should be checked daily for results:

    Place plucked hairs on the surface of the medium.

    Label with client/patient identification and the inoculation date.

    Leave the cap loose to allow oxygen for dermatophyte growth.

    Place in a warm, out-of-the-way area.

TREATMENT
Localized lesions

- Clip the affected areas to remove contaminated hair shafts. (Clippers will be contaminated.)
- Treat local areas twice daily with a topical antifungal medication. Continue treatment for 2 weeks after lesions clear. Recommended medications include the following:

    Conofite (Pitman-Moore)

    Tresaderm (MSD Agvet)

    Micatin Cream (Advanced Care)

    Monistat (Ortho)

    Lotrimin (Schering)

    Mycelex (Miles)

    Dilute Clorox solution

Generalized lesion

- Clip entire coat. Bathe animal in a medicated shampoo such as Nolvasan.
- Treat entire body with antifungal preparations 1 to 2 times weekly until cultures are negative. This may take 4 to 16 weeks or longer. Antifungal preparations include the following:

    Lyme Dyp (DVM)

    Nolvasan (Ft. Dodge)

    Betadine (Purdue Frederick)

    Clorox

- Oral therapy:
  Griseofulvin (microsize): 50 mg/kg orally q 24 h (Fulvicin U/F, Schering)
  Griseofulvin suspension (pediatric) (Ortho Pharmaceuticals): 20 to 50 mg/kg b.i.d. for 4 to 6 weeks. Griseofulvin may cause vomiting and diarrhea and is contraindicated in pregnant animals.
  Ketoconazole (Nizoral, Jansen): 10 mg/kg PO q 12 to 24 h with food. Side effects may include depression, anorexia, vomiting and diarrhea, elevated ALT, and jaundice.
  Microsporum canis vaccine (Fel-O-Vax MC-K, Ft. Dodge): Available for use in adult cats as an aid in treating the clinical signs of disease caused by *Microsporum canis*. The vaccine is given in three doses— two doses administered at 14-day intervals and the third given 28 days after the second dose. The vaccine *does not* eliminate *M. canis* from the animal (see package insert).

INFORMATION FOR CLIENTS

- This disease is contagious through contact with the organism.
- Fungal hairs remain infective on shed hairs of the animal for as long as 18 months. Environmental cleaning is a must to prevent reinfection. Carpets and furniture should be vacuumed weekly with the bag being discarded each time. Hard surfaces should be cleaned using a 1:10 Clorox solution or Nolvasan solution. Repaint surfaces not easily cleaned. Throw away toys and equipment not easily cleaned.
- Handle infected animals as little as possible.
- Some cats may be carriers of fungal infection while not exhibiting any clinical signs.
- See your doctor if lesions develop on family members.

PYODERMAS

Pyoderma is the term applied to bacterial infections involving the skin. Pyodermas may be primary or secondary, superficial or deep. The disease is recognized as part of several distinct clinical syndromes.

SUPERFICIAL PYODERMAS

Clinically seen diseases in this category include acute moist dermatitis ("hot spots"), impetigo, acne, and skin-fold pyodermas. The lesions typically involve only the superficial epidermis, with healing occurring without scarring. The disease is usually of short duration. The animal is rarely systemically ill. The skin around the lesion remains normal, whereas the affected portions may be ulcerated or traumatized by the animal.

ACUTE MOIST DERMATITIS ("HOT SPOTS")

This disorder occurs secondary to skin trauma (usually self-inflicted). Lesions appear rapidly as well-demarcated, red, moist, hot, and painful areas. The condition is common in heavy-coated, water loving breeds such as the Golden Retriever, Labrador Retriever, Newfoundlands, German Shepherds, and Saint Bernards. The incidence of the disease seems to be seasonal, being worse in the hot, moist summer months.

CLINICAL SIGNS
- Rapid appearance of red, hot, moist, painful patches
- Hair loss over the area
- Pruritus

DIAGNOSIS
- Visual inspection of the affected area reveals typical lesions.

TREATMENT
- Carefully clip the hair from the lesions. Clip area large enough to expose the edges of the lesion. If lesions are large, consider using sedation.
- Gently cleanse the skin using a medicated shampoo:
    Etiderm (Allerderm)
    ChlorhexaDerm (DVM)
- Apply topical medications to lesions twice daily. Avoid medications that dry or attract attention to the site, because this will increase self-trauma from licking or rubbing. Although topical medications are not frequently recommended, Gentocin spray has been of some use.
- Treat the original disease that induced the self-trauma to the skin (e.g., fleas, allergy).
- Cortisone and systemic antibiotics may speed healing:
    Prednisone: 1 mg/kg/day for 1 week
    Cephalexin: 22 mg/kg b.i.d.
    Enrofloxacin: 2.5 mg/kg b.i.d.
    Amoxicillin/clavulanic acid: 12.5 to 25 mg/kg b.i.d.

INFORMATION FOR CLIENTS
- Gentle cleansing of the area on a daily basis will speed recovery.
- Owners should wash their hands after treating an infected animal to prevent contamination with *Staphylococcus*. Although human infections are rare, the microorganism could present a danger to owners who are immunosuppressed.
- Lesions may be slow to heal.
- Owners should use an Elizabethan collar to prevent the animal from traumatizing the area.

IMPETIGO

This disease is seen most commonly in young dogs as a secondary infection related to malnourishment, debilitation, and poor hygiene. *Streptococcus* is the usual organism involved, although staphylococci are occasionally cultured from lesions. This disease is not contagious.

CLINICAL SIGNS
- Lesions are seen in young dogs.
- Lesions are commonly seen on the abdomen.
- Lesions include pustules that rupture to form honey-colored crusts.
- Lesions are nonpruritic and nonpainful.

DIAGNOSIS
- By physical appearance in a young animal
- Culture and sensitivity

TREATMENT
- Improve the animal's general health.
- Systemic antibiotics based on culture/sensitivity or an antibiotic with good gram-positive spectrum:
    Cephalexin: 22 mg/kg b.i.d.
    Enrofloxacin: 2.5 mg/kg b.i.d. (avoid use in young animals)
    Amoxicillin/clavulanic acid: 12.5 to 25 mg/kg b.i.d.
- Gently cleanse the lesions using an antibacterial shampoo such as Chlor-hexaDerm (DVM) or Etiderm (Allerderm): Use at 2- to 3-day intervals after initial cleaning.
- Topical antibiotic creams may be applied to lesions.

INFORMATION FOR CLIENTS

- This disease is not contagious.
- Programs for the elimination of parasites, improvement of the diet, and better sanitation should be implemented to improve the general health of the animal.
- Continue treatment for at least 2 weeks after lesions disappear.

ACNE

Although canine acne is fairly common in young (3 to 12 months of age), short-coated breeds, the disease presents few problems clinically. As dogs mature, lesions spontaneously heal. However, feline acne is clinically significant and often becomes a chronic problem. Acne can occur in cats of all ages.

CLINICAL SIGNS

- The chin may be swollen and painful to the touch.
- Owners may report seeing "dark spots" on the chin and be concerned about neoplasia.
- Large comedones (blackheads) may be present on the chin.
- Cats severely affected may be febrile.

DIAGNOSIS

- Characteristic appearance is diagnostic.
- Rule out other skin infections such as bite abscess.

TREATMENT

- Gently clip the hair on the chin.
- Cleanse with an antibacterial soap.
- Large comedones may require extraction under sedation.
- Clean daily with a human acne product such as Stridex pads (benzoyl peroxide).
- Provide systemic antibiotics for 14 to 21 days. The product should have a good gram-positive spectrum. (See Impetigo for antibiotic choices and doses.)

INFORMATION FOR CLIENTS

- This problem may become chronic.
- Daily cleaning of the chin may prevent further damage.

SKIN FOLD PYODERMAS

This type of pyoderma can occur wherever skin is plentiful: lips, facial folds, vulvar folds, and tail folds. The redundant tissue in these folds traps moisture and heat, whereas constant rubbing results in trauma and secondary infection. Facial folds may also present a danger to the cornea of the eye as the hairs on the fold rub across the surface of the cornea.

Skin fold pyodermas are usually a chronic problem requiring long-term medical treatment. Surgical removal of the excess skin is the only real cure.

DIAGNOSIS
- Presented with a commonly affected breed: Spaniels and Setters (lip fold), Pekinese and Pugs (facial fold), Boston Terriers and Pugs (tail fold), and very obese dogs of any breed (tail and vulvar folds).
- Report of a foul odor or discharge from the affected area can be diagnostic.
- Affected area will be moist, red, and ulcerated.

TREATMENT
- Relief of symptoms is the goal of treatment:
    Clip and clean the area.
    Dry the lesions. Topical drying agents may be used (e.g., cornstarch).
    Topical antibiotic ointments may be of some use.
- Surgical removal of the excess skin is the only real cure for the problem.
- Encourage weight reduction for obese animals through diet and exercise programs.

INFORMATION FOR CLIENTS
- This problem will require long-term medical treatment.
- The areas affected need to be kept dry and clean.
- Weight reduction is mandatory for those animals with tail-fold and vulvar-fold pyodermas.
- On dogs with facial folds, keep hair away from the eyes, and monitor the appearance of the cornea for signs of injury.

DEEP PYODERMAS

The deep pyodermas present a greater challenge clinically than do the superficial infections. Deep pyodermas tend to become chronic infections, often resistant to treatment. It has been speculated that these pyodermas may occur in animals with some degree of immunosuppression or allergy. A great many of these cases involve the microorganism *Staphylococcus intermedius,* previously known as *S. aureus,* which produces toxins and enzymes that cause severe tissue damage. Diseases seen clinically include juvenile pyoderma (puppy strangles), interdigital pyoderma (interdigital cysts), and generalized pyoderma (German Shepherd pyoderma). The clinical signs and treatments of all deep pyodermas are similar.

CLINICAL SIGNS
- Appearance of papules and pustules with crusting in characteristic locations is diagnostic.
- Dogs are often febrile.
- Draining fistula tracts with severe infection may exist.

DIAGNOSIS
- Clinical signs
- Culture and sensitivity
- Biopsy

TREATMENT
- Thorough and *gentle* daily cleaning of the infected areas
- Topical, water-based antibiotic creams, sprays, or solutions applied 2 to 4 times daily
- Systemic antibiotics chosen from the culture/sensitivity results or a good gram-positive spectrum drug. Therapy may be needed for 3 months or longer in many cases (see Superficial Pyoderma section for doses):
    Clavamox
    Enrofloxacin
    Cephalexin
- Staphylococcal bacterin given weekly:
    Staphoid-AB (Jensal)
    Staphage Lysate (Delmont Labs)

INFORMATION FOR CLIENTS
- The organism that is responsible for this disease is often drug resistant.
- Treatment may be prolonged and expensive in large breed dogs.
- Underlying conditions that predispose the animal to these infections

should be investigated. Diabetes mellitus and Cushing's disease are two conditions that may present as recurrent skin infections.
* Some animals will never get better.

ANAL GLANDS

The anal sacs create a special set of problems in companion animals. Three commonly seen anal sac problems are impaction, chronic infection, and rupture or abscessation. The anal sacs are located between muscle layers of the anus at the 4 and 8 o'clock positions. Each sac connects to the surface through a narrow duct. The sacs are lined with abundant sebaceous glands that produce an oily brown fluid that has a characteristic odor (foul smelling). When feces passes over the sacs, the sacs are compressed, expelling some of the fluid onto the surface of the fecal material. The odor of this fluid may have the function of social marking among dogs and cats. If the fluid produced becomes too thick or blockage of the duct occurs, the sacs will overfill. As water is reabsorbed from the fluid, the material dries out, resulting in impaction of the sac. Infections and impactions may result in anal sac rupture or abscessation. This condition is usually seen in small breed dogs.

CLINICAL SIGNS
* History of scooting the rear end across the floor or licking excessively at the perianal area
* Foul odor

DIAGNOSIS
* Digital palpation of distended anal sacs (may be performed rectally or externally)

TREATMENT
* Express contents of the distended sac (the dog may need sedation).
* Lavage infected sac with lactated Ringer's solution.
* Instill antibiotic ointment into the sac.
* Treat abscessed sacs aggressively with lavage and cleaning.
* Oral antibiotics may speed healing time.
* Chronically infected sacs should be surgically removed.
* *Remember:* Empty the opposite sac when you are treating a unilateral infection.

INFORMATION FOR CLIENTS

- Owners should be shown how to check their pet's anal sacs. If they request, demonstrate how to empty them.
- Scooting on the floor does not usually mean that the pet has worms.
- Blood under the tail may indicate a ruptured anal sac.
- These impactions and infections tend to recur.
- Cats can develop impactions, which may abscess.

TUMORS OF THE SKIN

The word *tumor* may be defined as a new growth of tissue characterized by progressive, uncontrolled proliferation of cells. Tumors can be *benign* (do no harm) or *malignant* (may result in death), localized or invasive. Malignant tumors usually consist of poorly differentiated cells that metastasize to other parts of the body and are usually invasive to surrounding tissues. Malignant tumors of the skin are usually *carcinomas* (those of epithelial origin) or *sarcomas* (those of connective tissue origin). An estimated 37% of canine tumors and 24% of feline tumors involve the skin.

Although no clear-cut cause of tumors has been found, certain trends are worth mentioning:

- Most skin tumors occur in older dogs (>6 years) and cats (>4 years).
- Younger dogs are more likely to acquire viral-induced tumors.
- Certain breeds, such as Boxers and Cocker Spaniels, seem to be more susceptible to tumor development.

Although the role genetics plays in the development of neoplastic disease (neoplasia) is still under investigation, neoplasia may be a result of a combination of events that allow a mass of unregulated cells to proliferate within the tissues of the body.

BENIGN SKIN TUMORS

HISTIOCYTOMAS

CLINICAL SIGNS

- Found almost exclusively in young dogs
- Small, buttonlike nodules, usually pink
- Usually hairless and may be ulcerated
- Found on the face, legs, lips, and abdomen
- Rapidly growing lesion

DIAGNOSIS

- General appearance
- Biopsy

TREATMENT

- Local surgical excision
- Many tumors regress spontaneously.

INFORMATION FOR CLIENTS

- These tumors are not malignant and do not metastasize.
- This tumor is not seen in cats.
- Lesions may regress spontaneously; however, surgical excision is the treatment of choice.

LIPOMA

CLINICAL SIGNS

- Obese, older dogs commonly affected.
- Females more commonly affected than males.
- Round or oval subcuticular masses
- Encapsulated and slow growing masses
- Lesions are soft.
- Many lesions are freely movable.

DIAGNOSIS

- Biopsy
- Fine needle aspiration (FNA) will provide a presumptive diagnosis. (A gray, greasy, mucoidlike substance is removed from the slide by the fixing step of staining.)

TREATMENT

- Surgical excision is the treatment of choice.
- Care should be taken to close the tissue space that results from removal of the mass.

INFORMATION FOR CLIENTS

- These masses rarely become malignant.
- They may recur after removal.
- A change in diet will probably not affect existing lipomas.
- These are benign tumors even though they may grow large.

PAPILLOMAS (WARTS)

CLINICAL SIGNS
- Young dogs are commonly affected.
- Lesion begins as a smooth, white, elevated lesion in the oral mucosa that develops into a cauliflower-like growth (may be few or multiple).
- Regression of the lesion may occur spontaneously.

DIAGNOSIS
- General appearance
- Biopsy

TREATMENT
- Surgical excision of large masses may stimulate regression of others.
- Autogenous vaccines can be made by grinding tumor tissue (1 : 4 weight to volume) in 0.5% phenol. Inject 1 to 5 ml intradermally weekly for 3 weeks.
- Lesions will usually regress with no treatment.

INFORMATION FOR CLIENTS
- This disease is caused by a DNA virus.
- Disease may last as long as 21 weeks or more.
- Cats are not affected.
- Older dogs are resistant.
- This disease usually regresses spontaneously, and adult animals become immune for life.

SEBACEOUS CYSTS

CLINICAL SIGNS
- May occur in dogs of any age or sex. The cysts are more common in Cocker Spaniels.
- Cysts are encapsulated, round, and fluctuate on palpation. When compressed, they may exude a gray, cheeselike material.
- Cysts slowly enlarge and may spontaneously rupture.
- Cysts may be found on the back, legs, chest, and neck of the animal.

DIAGNOSIS
- Characteristic contents of the cyst
- Histology of cyst wall

TREATMENT
- Surgical removal of *entire* encapsulated cyst

INFORMATION FOR CLIENTS
- These growths are formed by degenerative changes in the glandular area surrounding the hair follicle.
- These are benign growths.
- Surgical removal will cure the problem.
- These lesions are usually slow growing.
- Dogs may have multiple lesions at varying times, especially in breeds that are predisposed to this problem.

MALIGNANT SKIN TUMORS

BASAL CELL CARCINOMA

CLINICAL SIGNS
- Basal cell carcinoma is a common tumor of adult animals.
- A single, discrete lesion that is round, firm, and often ulcerated is found.
- This lesion is most commonly found on the head (around the eyes), ears, lips, neck, and legs.
- These lesions are slow growing.

DIAGNOSIS
- Biopsy

TREATMENT
- Wide surgical excision

INFORMATION FOR CLIENTS
- These tumors rarely metastasize.
- Local recurrence after surgery is possible.
- A less favorable prognosis exists if there are multiple lesions.

FIBROSARCOMAS (NOT VACCINE INDUCED)

CLINICAL SIGNS
- Older dogs are affected.
- Face, legs, and mammary glands are the most common sites.

- Tumors range in size, feel firm but rubbery on palpation, are unencapsulated, and feel adhered to underlying tissues.

DIAGNOSIS
- Biopsy

TREATMENT
- Wide surgical excision is necessary, and recurrence is common.

INFORMATION FOR CLIENTS
- Generally the prognosis for this disease is poor because the tumors are very invasive and metastasize readily.
- Recurrence is common.
- Other therapies such as radiation and chemotherapy are not usually effective.
- Wide surgical excision may require amputation of the limb.

FELINE FIBROSARCOMAS (VACCINE INDUCED)

Until the late 1980s this disease was unrecognized in cats. During that time a killed rabies vaccine and the feline leukemia vaccine became available to practitioners. The incidence of vaccination-related tumors began to increase, and within the last few years the incidence has risen to between 1:1000 and 1:10,000 vaccinated cats. With an estimated 20 million vaccines administered to pet cats throughout the world, this tumor development has become a significant problem for feline practitioners and owners. These tumors are rapidly developing, highly invasive, and malignant. They occur at the site of vaccination, usually within 4 to 6 weeks after the vaccine has been given. After routine surgical removal, they often recur. By the time many owners act, it is too late for the cat. In an effort to prevent or reduce the incidence of this disease, the Vaccine-Associated Sarcoma Task Force has issued the following guidelines for feline vaccination:

1. Use single-dose vaccines whenever possible. Intranasal vaccines should be chosen when available. Never vaccinate between the shoulder blades.
2. Rabies vaccine should be given as low on the *right* rear leg as possible, leukemia vaccine low on the *left* rear leg, and the distemper combinations on the *right* shoulder.
3. Any swelling not resolved within 6 weeks should be removed by radical surgical excision.

CLINICAL SIGNS
- Swelling over the site of a recent vaccination in a cat
- Rapidly growing, firm, often elongated mass

DIAGNOSIS
- Biopsy or needle aspiration may confirm suspicion.

TREATMENT
- Radical surgical excision, which may involve limb amputation, is the treatment of choice.

INFORMATION FOR CLIENTS
- This disease has a poor prognosis if not detected early and treated aggressively.
- Some individual cats or breeds of cats may be genetically at risk for this disease.
- Inflammatory lumps do develop over vaccine sites in many cats; however, they usually disappear within 1 to 2 weeks. If the lump does not resolve in 4 to 6 weeks, see your veterinarian.

❶ TECH ALERT
The vaccine most often suspected of causing these tumors has been the adjuvant rabies vaccine containing aluminum. Newer nonadjuvant rabies vaccines are on the market and should be used when possible.

MAST CELL TUMORS

CLINICAL SIGNS
- Isolated, firm nodules in the skin. About 50% are found on the rear legs, perineum, or external genitalia.
- Tumors may be ulcerated and edematous.
- These tumors are usually seen in dogs >6 years; cats >10 years.
- Siamese and males are usually predisposed.
- Lesions may appear crusty in cats.
- When crusts are removed, ulcerated surfaces are exposed.

DIAGNOSIS
- Biopsy

- Impression smears may demonstrate mast cell granules for presumptive diagnosis.

TREATMENT
- Surgical excision with a lymph node exam to rule out metastasis
- Chemotherapy (using the following drugs):
    Vinblastine: 2 mg/m^2 once weekly
    Cytoxan: 50 mg/m^2 daily q 4 days
    Prednisolone: 40 mg/m^2 daily for 1 week
- Prednisolone: 2.2 mg/kg PO q 24 h for 14 days, then ½ that dose for 14 days, then ½ dose q 48 h for 5 months
- Radiation and cryosurgery
- Cimetidine: 4 mg/kg q 6 h in cases of lymph node involvement or gastric ulceration or irritation
- Premedication with Benadryl 2.2 mg/kg IM has been recommended to block the histamine release caused by manipulation of the tumor at surgery.

INFORMATION FOR CLIENTS
- These tumors do not usually metastasize; however, up to 30% may metastasize.
- The prognosis depends on the amount of cell differentiation within the tumor. In dogs the survival times range from 18 to 51 weeks; in cats the lesions are usually benign.
- Recurrence at the surgical site is possible.
- A virus may cause these tumors.

MELANOMA (BENIGN OR MALIGNANT)

CLINICAL SIGNS
- Benign lesions are usually small, slow-growing hairless growths with dark pigmentation.
- Malignant growths are usually large, dome-shaped sessile growths of varying pigmentation.
- Tumors most commonly occur in the highly pigmented tissues of the canine (oral, skin, and digits).

DIAGNOSIS
- Biopsy

TREATMENT
- Surgical resection

INFORMATION FOR CLIENTS
- Tumors of the oral cavity and digits tend to be malignant.
- These tumors metastasize readily.
- Owing to early metastasis, the prognosis is often poor.
- Recurrence after surgery is common.
- In dogs with small lesions, median survival time is 12 months (54% are dead within 2 years). With large lesions, survival time is 4 months (100% are dead within 2 years).

PERIANAL TUMORS (ADENOMAS AND ADENOCARCINOMAS)

CLINICAL SIGNS
- Adenomas are most commonly seen in male dogs >8 years old.
- Carcinomas occur with equal frequency in males and females.
- Lesions are small, slow-growing, single or multiple lumps close to the anus.
- Lesions are frequently ulcerated, and owners may report seeing blood under the tail.
- Cocker Spaniels, Beagles, Samoyeds, and German Shepherds seem predisposed to these tumors.

DIAGNOSIS
- Clinical appearance and location
- Biopsy

TREATMENT
- Complete surgical excision is recommended.
- Castration aids in preventing recurrence of adenomas.
- Radiation and cryosurgery are both effective in treating these tumors.

INFORMATION FOR CLIENTS
- Castration of the intact male dog is highly recommended to prevent recurrence of adenomas.
- Adenomas rarely become malignant.
- Adenocarcinomas are usually highly invasive to surrounding tissue.

- Without a biopsy, it may be difficult to distinguish an adenoma from an adenocarcinoma.

Squamous Cell Carcinoma

CLINICAL SIGNS
- Older dogs and cats (>9 years of age)
- Lesions seen on the head, ears, oral cavity, nose, and neck of cats; trunk, toes, and scrotum of dogs (nonpigmented areas).
- Tumor appears as a raised, ulcerated, cauliflower-like mass with a necrotic odor.
- Affected animals have a history of being "sun bathers."

DIAGNOSIS
- Biopsy

TREATMENT
- Surgical excision
- Cryosurgery
- Radiotherapy (photodynamic therapy)

INFORMATION FOR CLIENTS
- These tumors occur most frequently in sun-damaged skin.
- Most tumors are locally invasive, but slow to metastasize.
- Recurrence after surgery is common.
- Preventing chronic exposure to the sun will prevent the development of the tumors.
- The degree of malignancy determines the prognosis, especially in cats whose poorly differentiated tumors have a poor prognosis.

DISEASES OF THE eight MUSCULOSKELETAL SYSTEM

The musculoskeletal system is responsible for movement and shape in all animals. Animals must be able to move, find food, seek shelter, and escape predators to survive. Without a rigid frame (the skeleton), flexible articulations (joints), and a system of pulleys (muscles, tendons, and ligaments), we would all be little more than lumps of tissue. The integration of these systems provides *movement*—one of the basic characteristics of life.

Disruption of the musculoskeletal system can occur as a result of the following:

- Trauma—fractures, ligament ruptures
- Degenerative disease—osteochondritis dissecans (OCD), degenerative joint disease (DJD), nonunited anconeal process
- Inflammation—myositis, panosteitis
- Poor conformation—luxating patella
- Neoplasia

Any disease or malfunction of this system compromises the animal's ability to maintain homeostasis with its environment.

LONG BONE FRACTURES

At least three fourths of long-bone fractures occur as a result of motor vehicle accidents. Other causes include indirect violence, bone disease, or repeated stress. These fractures may be classified as *open* (bone exposed through the skin) or *closed* (bone not exposed through the skin), *simple* or *comminuted* (splintered or fragmented), and *stable* or *unstable* (Fig. 8-1). The type of fracture and its location determine the best method of repair.

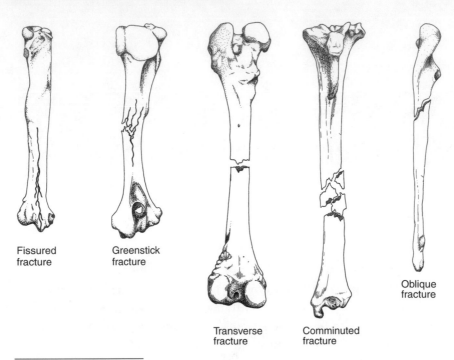

Fissured fracture

Greenstick fracture

Transverse fracture

Comminuted fracture

Oblique fracture

FIGURE 8-1. Common traumatic fractures. (From Christenson DE: *Veterinary medical terminology*, Philadelphia, 1997, WB Saunders.)

The job of the veterinary technician is to quickly assess the patient, especially in the case of motor vehicle accidents. After treatment for shock, hemorrhage, and soft tissue trauma, the possibility of fractures should be addressed. Technicians should always be aware that fractures might exist. They should take care when moving the animal, protect any areas of suspected fractures with support bandages if possible, and be careful not to make the injury worse by restraint methods or handling when obtaining radiographs.

CLINICAL SIGNS
- History of trauma
- Pain or localized tenderness
- Lameness
- Deformity of the bone
- Loss of function
- Crepitus
- Localized swelling or bruising

DIAGNOSIS

- Radiographs, at least two views, are required to diagnose and character-ize the fracture.
- Radiographs of the opposite limb may be of use for comparison.

TREATMENT

- Reduction and fixation of the fracture should be accomplished as soon as the patient is stable.

METHODS OF FIXATION

- *Splints*:
    A mold of material that surrounds the affected part is placed to hold the fracture segments in the reduced position while healing occurs.
    Use is usually limited to limbs.
    Make sure to use adequate padding to prevent the split from causing soft tissue injury.
    Keep the splint dry, and restrict activity.
    Evidence of problems with the splint include a foul odor, swelling, pain, fever, chewing at the splint, and generalized depression.
- *Casts*:
    Casts are made of plaster of Paris or other rigid, moldable material.
    Their function is similar to splints.

⊕ TECH ALERT

Casts and splints may not prevent rotation or overriding of fracture pieces and may result in delayed healing or nonunion in some fractures.

- *Intramedullary (IM) pins*:
    Provide good rigidity to fracture site (Fig. 8-2)
    May be used in combination with other methods to prevent rotation
    Usually require removal after the fracture has healed
    Must be inserted under sterile conditions
    Promote healing (adult dogs) in 7 to 12 weeks
- *Bone plates*:
    Work well on most long bone fractures, particularly in large dogs or a semidomesticated species
    Should always be removed after healing is complete. However, most are left in place unless they break, interfere with normal bone growth in young animals, or become irritating or infected.

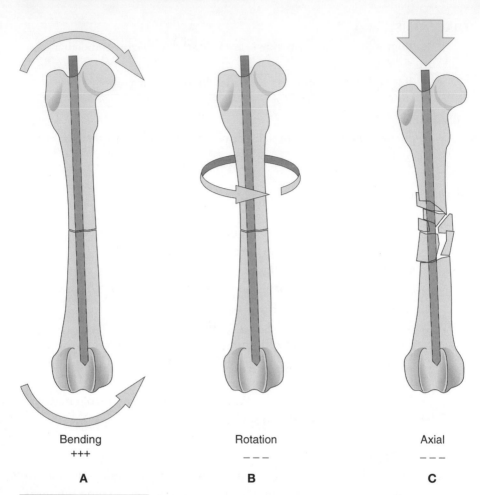

FIGURE 8-2.   A, The biomechanical advantage of intramedullary pins is that they are equally resistant to bending loads applied from any direction because they are round. **B** and **C,** Biomechanical disadvantages of intramedullary pins include poor resistance to rotational or axial (compressive) loads and lack of fixation (interlocking) with bone. (From Fossum TW: *Small animal surgery,* ed 2, St Louis, 2002, Mosby.)

Can usually be removed after bone union in adult dogs (5 to 12 months)

Require specialized instrumentation and surgical technique for correct application (Fig. 8-3)

Provide an early return to function

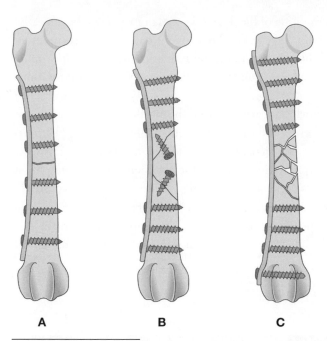

FIGURE 8-3.   Functions of a bone plate. **A,** Compression plate. **B,** Neutralization plate. **C,** Buttress plate. (From Fossum TW: *Small animal surgery,* ed 2, St Louis, 2002, Mosby.)

INFORMATION FOR CLIENTS

- Activity must be restricted while the bone is healing. Leash walking and cage rest may be required for 5 to 8 weeks.
- Report any evidence of drainage, swelling, or heat in the affected limb.
- Bone plates and IM pins are stronger than the surrounding bone, and refracture of the bone may occur in some cases. Report any change in use of the limb.
- Follow-up radiographs are required to assess healing. Surgery may be required to remove the pin or plate after healing has been completed.
- Some animals suffer cold sensitivity to plates and pins. If this occurs, the plates and pins may need to be removed.

CRUCIATE LIGAMENT INJURY

The *anterior* and *posterior cruciate ligaments* are intraarticular structures that help stabilize the stifle joint. Rupture of the cranial cruciate ligament is possibly the most common injury to the stifle of the dog and is a major cause of degenerative joint disease in the stifle joint (Fig. 8-4). The ligament may rupture completely, resulting in gross instability of the joint, or it may tear, producing minor instability. Both injuries result in degenerative changes within the joint within a few weeks.

Cruciate ligament injuries are usually seen in middle-age, obese, inactive animals that suddenly hyperextend their stifle joint while exercising. Rupture may also occur in animals engaged in athletic endeavors (such as racing or jumping), resulting in a traumatic injury to the ligament. There may be an occult degenerative process present in the former group of animals that predisposes the ligament to atraumatic rupture. In both groups, rupture of the opposite cruciate ligament often occurs within a year after injury to the first ligament. Approximately 50% of dogs with ligament rupture also demonstrate meniscal injury.

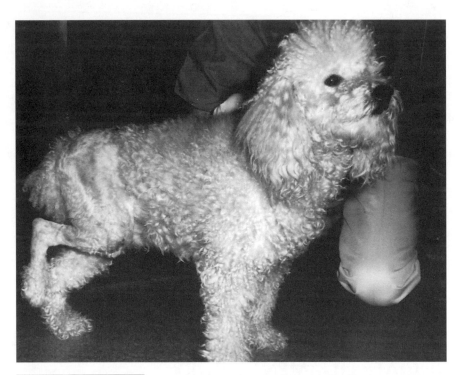

Figure 8-4. Poodle with rupture of the cranial cruciate ligament. The affected limb is held with the stifle in a flexed position and the paw off the floor. This is typical of (acute) stifle injuries. (From Olmstead ML: *Small animal orthopedics,* St Louis, 1995, Mosby.)

Treatment of this type of injury involves removal of the damaged tissue and stabilization of the joint. Many repair techniques have been reported; the choice of technique is usually based on the size of the dog, the activity level required by the animal, and the skill of the surgeon.

CLINICAL SIGNS

- Middle-age, obese animals or highly active, athletic animals are commonly affected.
- Injury occurs infrequently in cats.
- Animal demonstrates non–weight bearing on rear leg or appears to be in pain when affected leg is used.
- Tibia usually rotates internally when the animal tries to bear weight.
- If the injury is recent, the joint may show effusion (swelling).
- Generally the problem is acute in onset.

DIAGNOSIS

- Demonstration of a positive *cranial drawer movement.* (The tibia abnormally slides forward with respect to the femoral condyles.) The animal may need to be sedated to demonstrate this instability.
- Tibial compression test: The tibia moves forward with respect to the femur when the hock is flexed in the proper manner.
- Radiographs may show cranial displacement of the tibial plateau or a bony avulsion at the tibial attachment of the ligament.

TREATMENT

- Many methods of treatment can be found in the literature. The most successful techniques involve surgical stabilization of the stifle joint. In all cases, damaged tissue must be removed from the joint before stabilization.

EXTRAARTICULAR STABILIZATION TECHNIQUES

- These are most successful in animals weighing less than 15 kg.
- Suture material is placed around the caudal fabellae and through a tunnel in the tibial crest to stabilize the joint.
- Imbrication of the joint capsule and the lateral and medial muscle fascia is performed to "tighten" the joint.

INTRAARTICULAR STABILIZATION TECHNIQUE

- "Over-the-top" patellar tendon graft uses a strip of the patellar tendon to replace the cranial cruciate ligament.

- Tibial plateau leveling osteotomy prevents the tibia from moving forward against the pull of the hamstring muscles.
- The surgical techniques mentioned, among others, can be found in most veterinary orthopedic surgical texts. No matter which technique is chosen, the goal is always the same—to stabilize the joint and decrease the development of degenerative joint disease.

INFORMATION FOR CLIENTS

- The pet requires restricted exercise for the first 3 to 4 weeks after surgery. Restricted exercise means cage rest with leash walking for elimination.
- You may gradually increase exercise between 4 and 8 weeks after surgery.
- Your pet may return to full exercise between 8 and 12 weeks after surgery.
- The opposite cruciate frequently ruptures within 1 year after the first rupture.
- Weight reduction will benefit the obese animal.
- Even if surgical stabilization is performed, the animal will have some degenerative changes in the joint (arthritis) as it ages. Your pet may require treatment with antiinflammatory medication if lameness and pain occur.

PATELLAR LUXATIONS

Patellar luxations occur frequently in dogs and occasionally in cats. They may be divided into several classes:
- Medial luxation—toy, miniature, large breeds
- Lateral luxation—toy, miniature breeds
- Medial traumatic luxations—any breed
- Lateral luxation—large, giant breeds

MEDIAL LUXATION OF TOY, MINIATURE, AND LARGE BREEDS

These luxations occur early in life and are not related to trauma. They are often called "congenital" because they are usually the result of anatomic deformities. Approximately 75% to 80% of patellar luxations are medial displacements.

Anatomic derangements that predispose an animal to medial luxations include medial bowing of the distal third of the femur, shallow trochlear sulcus and a poorly developed medial ridge, medial torsion of the tibial tubercle, or medial bowing of the proximal tibia. Over time these derangements put added stress on the cranial cruciate ligaments, predisposing 15% to 20% of them to rupture.

Surgery is required to correct these problems. The technique chosen will depend on the degree of displacement and the degree of rotation present.

CLINICAL SIGNS

- Neonates or young puppies with abnormal hind limb function
- Young to mature animals with abnormal or intermittent gait problems are predisposed to this condition.
- Older animals with a sudden rear leg lameness are predisposed to this condition.

LATERAL LUXATION IN TOY AND MINIATURE BREEDS

This type of luxation is seen later in life as the soft tissues in the stifle begin to break down. The lateral deviations produce more functional disruption than the medial luxations.

CLINICAL SIGNS

- Acute development of lameness often associated with trauma or strenuous exercise is often seen.
- Knock-kneed stance is seen in some cases.
- If bilateral, animal may be unable to stand.

COMBINED MEDIAL AND LATERAL LUXATIONS OR MEDIAL LUXATIONS FROM TRAUMA

These conditions occur infrequently in small animals.

LATERAL LUXATION IN LARGE AND GIANT BREEDS

This type of problem is seen in the same breeds affected by hip dysplasia. Abnormal conformation at the hip results in a medial rotation of the femur and lateral displacement of the patella.

CLINICAL SIGNS
- The condition is usually bilateral.
- Animals affected are frequently between 5 and 6 months of age.
- Cow-hocked (external tibial rotation) gait is a clinical sign.
- Foot twists laterally when weight bearing.

DIAGNOSIS
- Palpation is used to test the ability to luxate the patella while the knee is flexed.
- Radiographs indicate anatomic deformity and patellar displacement.

TREATMENT
- Surgical correction is the treatment of choice. Methods range from mild soft tissue techniques to bone reconstruction. Usually both knees are corrected at the same time.

SOFT TISSUE TECHNIQUES
- Overlap of lateral or medial retinaculum
- Fascia lata overlap
- Patellar and tibial antirotational sutures
- Quadriceps release

BONE RECONSTRUCTION
- Trochleoplasty
- Transposition of the tibial tubercle
- Osteotomy or arthrodesis (joint fusion)

GOAL
- The goal of all surgical correction is to stabilize the stifle and return the patella to its functional position within the joint (and to keep it there). Combinations of several techniques may be required in some animals to achieve stability.

INFORMATION FOR CLIENTS
- After surgery, limit exercise for 2 to 3 weeks. Especially prevent jumping.
- A support bandage may be placed on the knee for 10 to 14 days to protect the surgical site. It should be kept dry.

- Aspirin or other antiinflammatory drugs can be used for pain.
- Physiotherapy such as swimming or passive flexion-extension of the joint (20 to 30 times four times daily) can be of benefit in animals that are reluctant to bear weight on the leg.
- The animal will probably have some degenerative changes in the joint later in life.

HIP DYSPLASIA

Dysplasia is one of the most prevalent disorders of the canine hip although it is rarely seen in animals weighing less than 11 to 12 kg. However, it has been reported in the occasional toy or small breed dog. The disease is complex, and the following factors have been identified as contributing to the development of hip dysplasia:

- Genetic predisposition (polygenic)
- Environment and dietary factors
- A disparity between muscle mass and the developing skeletal system
- Failure of the soft tissues of the hip to maintain joint congruity between the surfaces of the hip joint, resulting in bony changes within the joint

Hip dysplasia is a dynamic process and is often defined as a congenital, bilateral, degenerative joint disease, or as hip laxity. Any view of the disease is only a point along the progression of symptoms. The disease can be separated into *acetabular hip dysplasia* and *femoral hip dysplasia.*

ACETABULAR HIP DYSPLASIA

Most cases of dysplasia are of the acetabular form. This type is characterized by excessive slope of the dorsal rim of the acetabulum and the changes that result. Failure of the femoral head to press correctly into the developing acetabular cup results in damage to the dorsal rim. Osteophyte formation and damage to the joint capsule result in an unstable, painful joint.

FEMORAL HIP DYSPLASIA

In this form of dysplasia the femoral neck is shortened, decreasing the coverage by the acetabular rim and disrupting the congruity of the joint surfaces. In some cases the femur may be rotated. The joint lacks support from the acetabulum, which leads to osteophyte formation and joint capsule damage with joint instability.

CLINICAL SIGNS

- Clinical signs may vary with the age of the patient.
- Young dogs between 5 and 8 months of age and mature animals with chronic disease are predisposed to this condition.
- Difficulty in rising and stiffness that diminishes as the animal warms up on exercise are commonly seen.
- Pain is elicited on palpation of dorsal pelvic area or over hip joint.
- In older dogs you may see lameness, a waddling gait, and atrophy of the thigh muscles.
- Young dogs that are severely affected may be reluctant to stand or move.

DIAGNOSIS

- Radiographic confirmation of the disease is essential. The technician is referred to current radiology texts for positioning techniques.
- The Orthopedic Foundation for Animals (OFA) has established 7 grades of dysplasia:
    Excellent—nearly perfect conformation
    Good—normal for age and breed
    Fair—less than ideal but within normal limits
    Near normal—borderline conformation
    Mild dysplasia—minimal deviation with slight flattened femoral head and subluxation
    Moderate dysplasia—shallow acetabulum, flattened femoral head, poor joint congruency
    Severe dysplasia—complete dislocation of the hip with flattening of the acetabulum and femoral head
- For OFA certification, dogs should be radiographed after reaching 2 years of age. Any dog with clinical signs should be radiographed under anesthesia or sedation.

TREATMENT

CONSERVATIVE

- Moderate exercise
- Weight control
- Antiinflammatory medications, such as the following:
    Rimadyl: 2.2 mg/kg b.i.d.
    Aspirin (buffered): 25 mg/kg b.i.d.

Prednisone: 0.5 mg/kg daily, decreasing to level that keeps animal comfortable
- Nutriceuticals, such as the following:
  Adequan
  Cosequin

SURGICAL

- Femoral head ostectomy (FHO) (Fig. 8-5). Removal of the femoral head decreases pain that results from physical contact between the bone surface of the femur and the acetabulum. Removal allows formation of a "false joint" from the surrounding soft tissues. Vigorous exercise is required postoperatively to increase muscle strength and limb function. Swimming, walking, or running should be adequate to build muscle strength. Short periods of exercise (5 to 10 minutes t.i.d.) can gradually be lengthened (10 minutes q.i.d.) as the animal gains strength. Nonsteroidal antiinflammatory drugs can be used during rehabilitation. The operated limb may be slightly shorter than the opposite leg, and occasional lameness may be seen especially in larger dogs. This is not the suggested treatment for athletic dogs requiring complete return to normal joint function. It may take up to 1 year before optimal function returns to the limb.
- Total hip replacement (Fig. 8-6). This is the most effective way to give the patient a functional, nonpainful joint. The procedure replaces the femoral head and neck along with the acetabular cup. A cobalt chrome shaft and head are implanted into the femoral shaft and placed into an artificial acetabular cup. The advantages of this surgical procedure are as follows:
  Dogs achieve near-normal hind limb function approximately 95% of the time.

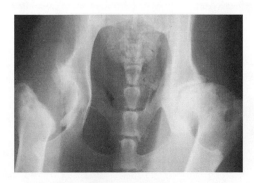

FIGURE 8-5. Radiograph of a dog after femoral head ostectomy. Note complete removal of the femoral neck. (From Fossum TW: *Small animal surgery,* ed 2, St Louis, 2002, Mosby.)

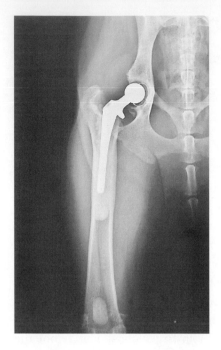

FIGURE 8-6. Radiograph of a dog after total hip replacement. Note the radiopaque cement mantel surrounding the femoral and acetabular prostheses. (From Fossum TW: *Small animal surgery,* ed 2, St Louis, 2002, Mosby.)

Patients achieve full range of motion in the joint and are pain free. Patients have a quick return to function.

- Pelvic osteotomy: A triple osteotomy of the pelvis allows rotation of the dorsal acetabular rim to provide increased coverage to the femoral head. Although technically difficult, the surgery provides for good return of function with minimal osteoarthritis.

INFORMATION FOR CLIENTS

- Dogs intended for breeding should have their hips radiographed after 2 years of age.
- Dogs may develop signs of dysplasia early in life.
- This is a progressive disease, and degeneration of the joint continues throughout the life of the pet.
- Weight loss and moderate exercise can reduce the pain felt by the animal.
- Puppies born to hip dysplasia–free parents *may* develop dysplasia.
- Surgery is the only cure for the disease.
- This condition is usually not seen in cats or small breed dogs.

LEGG-CALVE-PERTHES DISEASE (AVASCULAR NECROSIS)

This disease involves a noninflammatory aseptic necrosis of the femoral head and neck and is primarily a disease of small breed dogs. Although the exact cause is unknown, some vascular compression along with hormone activity has been suggested.

In affected dogs, the femoral head and neck undergo necrosis and deformation. The articular cartilage cracks and collapses due to the collapse of the subchondral bone. The result of these changes is pain and loss of joint congruity. Toy breeds and terriers are most commonly affected.

CLINICAL SIGNS
- Young dogs between 5 and 8 months of age are predisposed to this condition.
- Irritability and chewing at the hip or flank area is seen.
- Pain is a clinical sign.
- Atrophy of the muscles of the hip is noticeable.
- There is a gradual onset of lameness.

DIAGNOSIS
- Radiographic signs include decreased bone density in the femoral head and neck area, flattened femoral head, and osteophytes in the joint.

TREATMENT
- Excision arthroplasty removes the femoral head and neck. Postoperative treatment requires early, active use of the limb. As early as 2 weeks after surgery, animals should be encouraged to swim or run. Return to pain-free function may occur as early as 30 days postoperatively.

INSTRUCTIONS FOR CLIENTS
- Animals may have both hips involved.
- There may be a genetic predisposition for the disease.
- Patients require frequent physical therapy during recovery (exercise and passive range-of-motion exercises).
- If both hips are diseased, the surgeries are usually performed 8 to 10 weeks apart, depending on the surgeon's preference.

OSTEOCHONDROSIS DISSECANS (OCD)

Osteochondrosis refers to the degeneration or aseptic necrosis of bone and cartilage followed by reossification. If the condition results in a dissecting cartilage flap with inflammatory joint changes, it is termed *osteochondrosis dissecans* (Fig. 8-7). The underlying defect in this disease is one of endochondral ossification. Failure of the lower layers of physeal or articular cartilage to mature into bone results in thickened cartilage that is prone to injury. If lack of ossification occurs at the physis, problems such as nonunited anconeal process or retained cartilage cores can occur. If it occurs at the articular surface, OCD may occur. The disease is seen in several joints (the shoulder, stifle, hock, and elbow). OCD of the scapulohumeral joint (shoulder) is most commonly seen. Failure of the articular cartilage to become cemented to the underlying bone

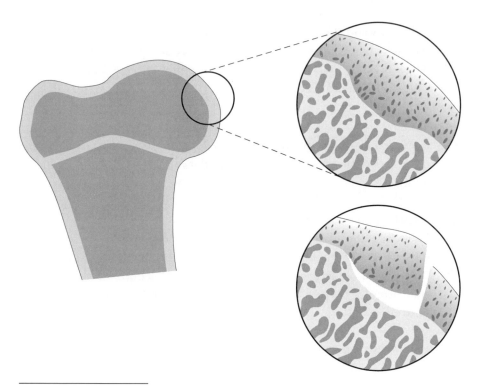

FIGURE 8-7.   Failure of endochondral ossification leads to cartilage thickening. Loss of chondrocytes deep in the cartilage layer produces a cleft and causes development of vertical fissures in the cartilage. These fissures eventually communicate with the joint, forming a cartilage flap. (From Fossum TW: *Small animal surgery,* ed 2, St Louis, 2002, Mosby.)

along with constant trauma during exercise results in the formation of a nonhealing cartilage flap. The presence of this flap produces lameness and osteoarthrosis.

CLINICAL SIGNS
- Lameness in large breed dogs (3 to 18 months of age) is a clinical sign.

DIAGNOSIS
- Radiographs reveal the cartilage flap with or without joint mice (loose cartilage pieces).

TREATMENT
- In early stages—rest and weight control
- If lame—surgical removal of the flap and/or mice

INFORMATION FOR CLIENTS
- A return to normal function occurs almost immediately after surgery.
- This is normally a disease of large breed dogs.
- This disease may have a hereditary component.

PANOSTEITIS (ENDOSTEOSIS, EOSINOPHILIC PANOSTEITIS)

This is a common disease that results in intermittent lameness in medium to large breed dogs. The average age of onset is 6 to 8 months. The lameness is usually acute, not associated with trauma, and may seem to the owner to shift from leg to leg. Male dogs are more commonly affected (66% of cases) with the German Shepherd breed being overrepresented.

The etiology of the disease is unknown but some causes may include viral infection, genetic predisposition, metabolic disease, and allergic or hormonal excess. Viral infection is thought to be the most likely cause. The disease affects the medullary bone marrow and the endosteal bone, resulting in degeneration of medullary marrow and thickening of the endosteal bone. Long bones such as the ulna, humerus, radius, femur, and the tibia are most commonly involved.

The disease is self-limiting and virtually all affected dogs return to normal within one year. During bouts of pain and lameness analgesics and nonsteroidal antiinflammatory drugs can be used to make the animal more comfortable.

CLINICAL SIGNS
- Intermittent lameness shifting from leg to leg
- Anorexia
- Fever
- Weight loss
- Reluctance to move

DIAGNOSIS
- Pain elicited on deep palpation of the long bone
- Radiology: Gray, hazy, patchy areas of increased radiodensity in the medullary cavity of the long bone

TREATMENT
- Analgesics and antiinflammatory drugs for pain:
  Aspirin: 25 mg/kg PO q 8 h
  Rimadyl: 2.2 mg/kg PO b.i.d.
  Phenylbutazone: 13 mg/kg PO t.i.d., then tapered (800 mg/day maximum dose)

INFORMATION FOR CLIENTS
- This disease is self-limiting and usually leaves no permanent damage.
- Drugs such as aspirin and phenylbutazone can cause gastric upset and ulceration in the dog. Report any vomiting of blood, blood in the stool, or lack of appetite.
- Flare-up of the disease is common, so animals may appear cured only to relapse. The disease is seldom seen in animals over 2 years of age.

LUXATIONS

Luxations of the hip are fairly common secondary to trauma in small animals. All luxations involve tearing of the joint capsule and round ligament. Specific signs vary depending on the location of the femoral head with respect to the acetabulum.

- *Craniodorsal*—the most common type. The leg appears shortened; the stifle rotates outward and the hock rotates inward.
- *Craniocaudal*—rare. The stifle rotates inward, the hock outward.
- *Ventral*—rare. The affected limb appears longer.

CLINICAL SIGNS
- History of trauma
- Acute lameness, non–weight bearing
- Possible swelling over the hip joint or in area dorsal to hip joint

DIAGNOSIS
- Radiographs can rule out other diseases such as femoral neck fractures, acetabular fractures, or Legg-Calve-Perthes disease. The presence of fractures or bone chips indicates a need for open surgical reduction of the dislocation.

TREATMENT
- Closed reduction (requires anesthesia): The femoral head is manually rotated and replaced back into the acetabulum using traction.
- Open reduction: The femoral head is surgically replaced into the acetabulum and the soft tissue structures are used to secure the reduction. The limb should be supported in an Ehmer sling for a minimum of 7 to 10 days; limit exercise for 3 weeks following removal of the sling.

INSTRUCTIONS FOR CLIENTS
- The prognosis will depend on the stability of the reduced joint and the amount of soft tissue injury.
- Pets may develop varying degrees of osteoarthritis after traumatic luxation.
- If the hip does not remain reduced, an FHO should be considered.

🜂 TECH ALERT
Luxations of other joints occur as a result of trauma. The goal of treatment is to return the joint to normal position and function. This is usually accomplished in a manner similar to that for the hip.

MYOPATHIES

Myopathies are diseases that affect muscle. Although there are many of these, the most commonly seen include *inflammatory myopathy, immune-mediated myopathy,* and *acquired myopathy.*

INFLAMMATORY MYOPATHIES

Bacterial myositis, a rarely occurring disease in the dog and the cat, typically occurs following a bite wound, trauma, or with contamination after surgical procedures. The most commonly involved microorganisms are *Staphylococcus* and *Clostridia* spp. Treatment should be based on culture and sensitivity results.

Protozoal myositis occurs when cysts are formed within the muscles of *Toxoplasmosis*-positive cats. Rupture of these cysts or immune response to their presence results in clinical signs of muscle *hyperesthesia*.

IMMUNE-MEDIATED MYOPATHIES

Polymyositis is an immune-mediated disease of muscles affecting dogs and cats. Middle-age, large breed dogs are most commonly affected. Weakness that gets worse with exercise, hyperesthesia on palpation, fever, and depression may all be signs of muscle involvement. Some dogs may have megaesophagus. Muscle atrophy may be seen with chronic cases. Diagnosis is most readily obtained through muscle biopsy; treatment involves prednisone, 2.2 mg/kg daily.

Masticatory muscle myositis, also known as *atrophic myositis* or *eosinophilic myositis,* involves the muscles of mastication in the dog. These muscles contain a special type of fiber (Type 2M), which has antigenic properties possibly shared with bacteria. Infections elsewhere in the body may incite an immune response affecting these muscle fibers. The masticatory muscles initially become swollen and painful. With chronic involvement, the muscles atrophy and fibrose. Glucocorticoids are the treatment of choice.

ACQUIRED MYOPATHIES

Feline polymyopathy occurs in cats of all ages, genders, and breeds. Hypokalemia results in cervical ventriflexion, periodic weakness, and muscle pain. These symptoms may occur concurrently with renal disease. Treatment involves supplementation of potassium and adjustment of diet.

CLINICAL SIGNS
- Muscle weakness, pain, swelling, or atrophy

DIAGNOSIS
- Clinical signs
- Muscle biopsy
- Serum chemistries (creatine kinase may be elevated)

TREATMENT
- Appropriate antibiotics if bacterial; antiprotozoal drugs if parasite related
- Glucocorticoids: 2.2 mg/kg daily (may be needed long term in some cases)

INFORMATION FOR CLIENTS
- Most animals show improvement with treatment.
- Treatment may be required for the life of the animal.
- Early intervention improves the prognosis.

TUMORS OF BONE

The diagnosis of bone cancer is devastating to the animal, the owner, and the veterinarian. There is a high incidence of bone cancer in pet animals, especially dogs. The onset of the disease is often acute, and the progression of signs rapid.

Approximately 8000 cases of bone cancer are seen in dogs each year. Of these, 85% to 90% involve osteosarcoma, a primary bone neoplasm. As with most cancers, the etiology of osteosarcoma is unknown. Studies suggest that a derangement of growth or differentiation of new bone at the metaphyses of long bones may result in tumor formation. The most common bones affected are the distal radius, proximal humerus, distal femur, and proximal tibia. The disease is most commonly seen in large breed, male dogs around 7 years of age. Most of these tumors show microscopic spread by the time they are diagnosed. Ninety percent of all diagnosed cases die despite treatment.

Primary bone cancer in cats is less common. As many as 90% of bone cancers seen in cats are osteosarcomas. Survival rates following amputation seem somewhat better than those for dogs.

CLINICAL SIGNS
- Lameness
- Weight loss
- Pain, especially over the affected bone
- Swelling in the affected limb

DIAGNOSIS
- Radiographs show mixed osteolysis, proliferation of bone, and periosteal reaction.

- Biopsy is required for diagnosis.
- Thoracic radiographs should be taken to rule out metastatic tumors.

TREATMENT
- Amputation of affected limb is required.
- Follow-up treatment with cisplatin or carboplatin can increase survival time.
- Radiation therapy can be provided for pain control.
- No recommended drug therapies exist for cats.

INFORMATION FOR CLIENTS
- This is a fatal disease.
- Survival times of up to 12 months may be achieved with aggressive treatment.
- Biopsy of the tumor is necessary to confirm the tumor type.
- Amputation is required to remove the primary tumor; however, it will not affect metastatic tumor cells elsewhere in the body.
- Drug therapy is expensive, and patients require laboratory monitoring to avoid bone marrow or renal toxicities from the treatment.

Diseases of the Nervous System

nine

The nervous system can be divided into two primary divisions, the *central nervous system (CNS)*, composed of the brain and the spinal cord, and the *peripheral nervous system (PNS)*, composed of the cranial nerves and the peripheral nerves that connect the outside sensory world to the brain.

The functional cell of both systems is the neuron, whose job is to transmit electrical impulses to and from the brain. Disease anywhere within the transmission system results in interruption of messages and clinical neurologic symptoms. The individual symptoms vary depending on the location of the lesion. For the purpose of this chapter, diseases will be divided into those of the brain, the spinal cord, and the peripheral nervous system.

BRAIN

TRAUMA

In small animal medicine, traumatic brain injuries are frequently encountered. The injuries generally have an acute clinical onset resulting from a traumatic experience (e.g., being hit by a car, having the head closed in a door, or falling). Injury to the brain from trauma can result from direct injury to the nervous tissues (primary event) or from secondary events, which intensify or worsen the neurologic damage and produce systemic derangements.

Primary events may produce disruption of fiber tracts, which cannot be repaired, or reparable cell damage, which is reversible.

Secondary events such as increased intracranial pressure (ICP), edema, hypoxia, and seizures occur as a result of the primary trauma. Increased ICP is caused by both edema and hemorrhage in or around the brain. Because the brain is encased in a nonflexible shell of bone (the skull), herniation of nervous tissue (primarily the brain stem) through the foramen magnum results.

Treatment of head trauma involves preventing or decreasing the secondary effects of trauma.

CLINICAL SIGNS
- History of trauma to the head
- Seizures
- Blood in ears, nose, oral cavity
- Ocular hemorrhage
- Loss of consciousness or a decrease in responses to external stimuli
- Signs of shock, cardiac arrhythmias, altered respiratory patterns, coma

DIAGNOSIS
- History and physical examination
- Serum chemistries to rule out metabolic problems
- Clinical rating scale for prognosis of trauma (Table 9-1)

TREATMENT
- Correct any metabolic derangements.
- Provide oxygen through mask or nasal canulla.
- Elevate the head.
- Administer osmotic agents to decrease cerebral edema:
  Mannitol (20%): 1 g/kg IV slow bolus
  Diuretics: Furosemide 0.7 mg/kg IV q 4 h
- Antiseizure medication if needed:
  Diazepam: 1 to 4 mg/kg divided into 3 or 4 doses
  Phenobarbital: 2.2 to 4.4 mg/kg IV or IM q 6 h
- Corticosteroids: Prednisolone sodium succinate 30 mg/kg IV

INFORMATION FOR CLIENTS
- Some brain damage is irreversible. If the animal survives, it may never return to "normal."
- In general, patients in a coma for longer than 48 hours do not survive.
- Deteriorating signs represent a worsening of the situation.

IDIOPATHIC VESTIBULAR DISEASE

This is an acute disorder of both dogs (middle age) and cats. In cats, the disease is seen most frequently during the late spring, summer, and early fall.

TABLE 9-1.   Clinical rating scale for evaluation of craniocerebral trauma (CCT)

CRITERIA	SCORE
MOTOR ACTIVITY	
Normal gait, normal reflexes	6
Hemiparesis, tetraparesis, or decorticate activity	5
Recumbent with intermittent extensor rigidity	4
Recumbent with constant extensor rigidity	3
Recumbent with intermittent extensor rigidity/opisthotonos	2
Recumbent, hypotonic with depressed-absent spinal reflexes	1
BRAIN STEM REFLEXES	
Normal pupillary light reflex (PLR) and oculovestibular reflexes (OVRs)	6
Slow PLR and normal to reduced oculovestibular reflexes	5
Bilateral/unresponsive miosis and normal to reduced OVRs	4
Pinpoint pupils and reduced to absent OVRs	3
Unilateral/unresponsive mydriasis and reduced to absent OVRs	2
Bilateral/unresponsive mydriasis and reduced to absent OVRs	1
LEVEL OF CONSCIOUSNESS	
Occasionally alert and responsive	6
Depressed/delirious, but capable of response to stimulus	5
Obtunded/stupor, but responds to visual stimuli	4
Obtunded/stupor, but responds to auditory stimuli	3
Obtunded/stupor, but responds to noxious stimuli	2
Comatose and unresponsive to noxious stimuli	1

TOTAL SCORE	PROGNOSIS
3-8	Grave
9-14	Poor to guarded
15-18	Good

From Fenner WR: Diseases of the brain. In Ettinger SJ, Feldman EC, editors: *Textbook of veterinary internal medicine,* ed 5, Philadelphia, 2000, WB Saunders.

Clinical signs involve loss of balance, nystagmus, disorientation, and ataxia. Many animals experience nausea early in the course of the disease. Animals stabilize rapidly, and clinical signs usually resolve in 3 to 6 weeks.

CLINICAL SIGNS
- Incapacitating loss of balance
- Nystagmus
- Disorientation
- Ataxia
- Vomiting
- Anorexia

DIAGNOSIS
- Clinical signs
- Blood work to rule out other diseases involving the nervous system
- Otic exam to rule out inner ear problem

TREATMENT
- Treatment is usually not recommended and does not alter the course of the disease.
- Supportive therapy and force feeding should be implemented.

● TECH ALERT

Steroids and antibiotics are used routinely to cover possible causes missed by physical exam and laboratory work.

- Confine the animal to prevent injury from falling.

NEOPLASIA

An enlarging tumor within the brain produces tissue compression and/or replaces normal neuronal tissue resulting in clinical signs that are *progressive*. Primary brain tumors are typically singular, but metastatic tumors or secondary brain tumors may be solitary or multiple in occurrence. Most tumors are metastatic by the time the patient is presented. The disease is typically seen in older animals.

CLINICAL SIGNS
- Signs reflect tumor location
- Seizures (typically increasing in frequency and severity)

- Endocrine derangements
- Presence or absence of vestibular signs
- Tremor, ataxia

DIAGNOSIS
- Systematic screening for primary tumors in other organs
    Blood work: CBC and serum chemistries
    Radiographs
- Cerebrospinal fluid (CSF) tap shows increased pressure, increased albumin, usually normal white blood cell count.
- Ophthalmic exam indicates optic nerve edema.
- CT scan or MRI provides the best chance of locating the lesion.

TREATMENT
TREATMENT OF THE TUMOR
- Surgical removal for superficial singular lesions (newer techniques may make deeper removal a possibility in the future)
- Radiation therapy
- Chemotherapy (lymphomas respond well, others are less responsive)

TREATMENT OF CLINICAL SIGNS
- Antiseizure medication: Phenobarbital 1 to 2 mg/kg PO b.i.d. to t.i.d.
- Corticosteroids: Prednisone 0.5 to 1 mg/kg s.i.d. to q.o.d.

INFORMATION FOR CLIENTS
- Unless the tumor can be removed surgically, medication will not cure the problem.
- Symptoms will gradually become more severe as the tumor grows in size.

IDIOPATHIC EPILEPSY

Idiopathic epilepsy is a syndrome characterized by repeated episodes of seizures for which there is no demonstrated etiology. The diagnosis is one of exclusion.

Idiopathic epilepsy is predominantly a disease in German Shepherds, Miniature and Toy Poodles, Saint Bernards, Cocker Spaniels, Beagles, Irish Setters, Golden Retrievers, and some mixed breeds. Seizures usually begin between 1 and 3 years of age. Affected animals may exhibit a short aura during which the animal may act abnormally. They may hide, seek companionship, vocalize, or exhibit other abnormal behaviors. Seizures are usually generalized in nature, lasting anywhere from 1 to 2 minutes. After the seizure, the animal is usually disoriented and occasionally blind. Seizures may occur singly or in clusters and may reoccur at fairly regular intervals. In some animals, inciting events such as excitement or estrus has been shown to precipitate seizure activity.

Although the cause of idiopathic epilepsy is unknown, a hereditary basis has been suggested.

CLINICAL SIGNS
- Seizures, often occurring at regular intervals
- Young animals typically affected
- Normal behavior between seizures

DIAGNOSIS
- CBC and serum chemistries to rule out hypocalcemia, hypoglycemia, infection, hepatic encephalopathy, lead poisoning
- Radiographs to rule out head trauma or hydrocephalus
- CT scan or MRI to rule out space-occupying lesions in the brain

TREATMENT
- Treatment should be directed at primary disease if one can be found.
- Initiate treatment if seizure frequency is more than once per month.
- Control seizure activity with phenobarbital: 2 mg/kg b.i.d. to t.i.d.

⊙ TECH ALERT
Drug takes 7 to 10 days to reach steady-state serum concentration in the body. If the animal continues to experience seizures after this time period, measure serum phenobarbital concentration 2 hours before and after dosing. If <20 µg/ml, slowly increase the dose by 10% to 20% until the concentration reaches 20 to 30 µg/ml.

- If seizures occur and phenobarbital concentration is adequate, add potassium bromide (KBr) 22 mg/kg s.i.d. with food.

STATUS EPILEPTICUS

Animals prone to seizures may exhibit status epilepticus, a medical emergency. Continual seizures for a prolonged period (>5 to 10 minutes) can lead to irreversible coma and death if not treated aggressively. Owners should be advised to seek emergency assistance if this situation develops.

CLINICAL SIGNS
- Prolonged, uninterrupted seizure activity

DIAGNOSIS
- History and clinical signs

TREATMENT
IMMEDIATE TREATMENT
- Diazepam: 2 mg IV (5-kg dog or cat); 5 mg IV (10-kg dog); 10 mg IV (20-kg dog). Can repeat 2 to 3 times over several minutes.
- Sodium pentobarbital IV to effect (not to exceed 15 mg/kg)
- Establish an airway and give oxygen.
- Place an IV catheter and start fluids to provide vascular access (TKO).
- Check blood glucose and calcium concentrations. Correct if necessary. Perform serum chemistries to rule out metabolic causes of seizure.
- Monitor body temperature. If >105° F, give a cool bath.
- If cerebral edema is suspected, give mannitol 2.2 g/kg IV and prednisolone sodium succinate 10 to 30 mg/kg IV.

MAINTENANCE THERAPY
- Phenobarbital: 2.2 to 4.4 mg/kg IV or IM q 6 h
- Initiate oral therapy if possible.

INFORMATION FOR CLIENTS
- This is an incurable disease.
- Even with treatment animals may have seizures. The goal of treatment is to decrease the frequency and severity of the seizures.
- Spaying or neutering the animal will prevent any hormonal influence on seizure activity.
- Medication will probably be required for the life of the pet. Missing doses or abruptly stopping medication will precipitate a seizure.
- Most animals with seizures can live a fairly normal life.
- Periodic monitoring of serum anticonvulsant concentration is required.
- Animals that remain seizure free for 6 to 9 months may have their medication dose slowly decreased until it may eventually be discontinued (in consultation with the veterinarian).

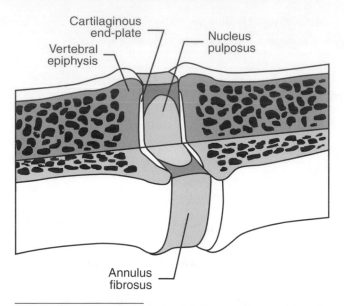

FIGURE 9-1.   The intervertebral disk is an elastic cushion between the adjacent vertebrae. This is a view of an intervertebral disk space showing relationships of the disk to the cartilaginous end-plates and epiphyses of the vertebrae.

SPINAL CORD

Just like the brain, the spinal cord is protected by a bony housing, the vertebral column. The spinal cord is located within the spinal canal, dorsal to the vertebral bodies. Between each of the vertebral bodies is a cushion known as the intervertebral disk. These disks are composed of an outer fibrous layer, the *annulus fibrosus,* and an inner gellike nucleus, the *nucleus pulposus.* Their presence allows a larger range of motion in the vertebral column and prevents the vertebral bodies from rubbing against each other (Fig. 9-1).

INTERVERTEBRAL DISK DISEASE

By far, one of the most common disorders involving the spinal cord of small animals is intervertebral disk disease. Disk protrusions can occur in all breeds of dog and occasionally in cats. It has been reported that 75% to 100% of all disks in chondrodystrophic breeds have undergone degenerative changes by 1 year of age. Disk protrusion or extrusion occurs most commonly in the cervical, caudal thoracic, and lumbar spine. Two types of herniations have been reported. Type 1 (common in younger dogs) involves acute rupture of the

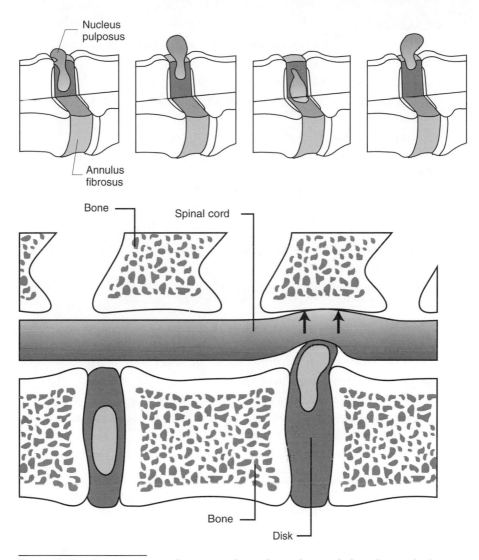

FIGURE 9-2. Various stages of a ruptured annulus and extruded nucleus, which may be degenerated, fibrotic, or even calcified.

annulus fibrosus and extrusion of the nucleus pulposus up into the spinal canal. In Type 2 (common in older [>5 years], large breed dogs) the extrusion occurs over a longer period of time, producing less acute and less severe clinical signs. The severity of spinal cord injury depends on the speed at which the disk material is deposited into the spinal canal, the degree of compression, and the duration of compression. Clinical signs may be related to the location of the lesion (Fig. 9-2).

CLINICAL SIGNS

- Apparent pain; presence or absence of motor or sensory deficits
- Acute onset (Type 1 usually)
- Paresis or paralysis that may be unilateral or bilateral
- Decreased panniculus reflex one to two vertebral spaces caudal to the actual lesion
- Altered deep pain response

DIAGNOSIS

- Age, breed, clinical signs, and history
- Complete neurologic exam
- Radiographs require anesthesia for proper positioning. Narrowed disk spaces at the location of the lesion may be seen. (C7-T1, T9-10, L7-S1 are normally narrow.)
- Myelogram is required for definitive location of the lesion.

TREATMENT
TYPE 1

- Medical treatment is recommended for animals with pain, with or without mild neurologic deficits:
    Strict confinement for a minimum of 2 weeks (cage rest)
    Corticosteroids injected for 1 to 2 days to decrease edema and inflammation
- Intensive nursing care: These animals require soft padding in the cage; some may require indwelling urinary catheters for expression of the bladder; some may need to be turned frequently to prevent pressure sores; and all animals should receive proper nutrition to promote healing.
- Surgical treatment should be reserved for animals with multiple episodes, ataxia, paresis or paralysis, and absence of deep pain:
    Fenestration, hemilaminectomy
    Decompression should be performed as soon as possible to prevent further damage to the cord.

TYPE 2

- Because of the slow progression of spinal compression accompanied by degeneration of spinal tissue, these dogs may improve initially on cortisone; however, surgery may fail to improve spinal function.

INFORMATION FOR CLIENTS

- Prevent excess weight gain in breeds prone to disk disease.
- Avoid having the animal stand on the hind legs or in any other position that strains the back.
- The prognosis for animals lacking deep pain for greater than 24 hours is poor.
- Animals lacking deep pain for less than 24 hours have a guarded to poor prognosis.
- The prognosis for animals having or regaining deep pain postsurgically is fair to good.
- Approximately 40% of animals treated medically had recurrence of disease with more severe signs.
- Animals with paresis or paralysis require intensive nursing care. They may need extensive home care while they are recovering.
- Severe damage to the spinal cord is not reparable at this time.

SPINAL CORD TRAUMA

Acute spinal cord injuries of the dog and cat usually result from motor vehicle accidents, gunshot wounds, or fights. The spinal cord trauma is sudden in onset and may be related to the velocity of cord compression, the degree of compression, and the duration of the compressive force. Signs of injury are typically nonprogressive, although they may worsen over the first 48 hours before stabilization. Injury may occur at a single or multiple levels within the spinal cord.

Blunt trauma to the spinal cord causes tissue injury through both "direct" and "indirect" mechanisms. Direct effects are due to primary disruption of neural pathways within the cord. Indirect effects are less well understood and include edema, hemorrhage, ischemia, lactic acidosis, inflammation, and neuronophagia by white blood cells. It seems that mechanical deformation of any type can trigger these secondary events within the spinal cord. Autodissolution of the cord may be seen as early as 24 hours after injury.

CLINICAL SIGNS

- History of trauma (affected animals usually have serious injury to other organ systems)
- Presence of the Schiff-Sherrington sign: Rigid hypertonicity of front legs, hypotonicity of the rear legs, normal reflexes, and pain percep-

tion caused by the release of inhibitory pathways along the spinal cord from L1-L7
- Lack of panniculus reflex caudal to lesion
- Paresis or paralysis

DIAGNOSIS
- Complete neurologic examination to localize the lesion
- Radiographs

ⓘ TECH ALERT

To prevent additional damage, limit manipulation of the spinal column while obtaining radiographs. Remember that the vertebral column may return to a normal position after trauma, hiding the original compressive event. A myelogram may be necessary to locate the actual sites of cord injury.

TREATMENT
MEDICAL TREATMENT
- Corticosteroids:
    Dexamethasone: 0.55 to 2.2 mg/kg IV
    SoluDelta Cortef: 132 mg/kg divided q 8 h
- Mannitol: 1 g/kg IV
- Dimethylsulfoxide (40%): 1 g/kg IV
- Treat other life-threatening injuries with IV fluids, oxygen; monitor heart rhythms and urine production
- Strict confinement for 6 to 8 weeks for mild fractures or dislocation (showing few clinical signs)

SURGICAL TREATMENT
- Treatment should be instituted within 2 hours of trauma if possible. Surgical treatment should be considered in cases of severe paresis or paralysis, myelographic evidence of continuing cord compression, or worsening clinical signs.
- Laminectomy should be performed at all sites of cord compression.
- Stabilization of vertebral column fractures or subluxations must be performed.
- Removal of all bone fragments or disk material from the spinal canal must be accomplished.

- A durotomy may be required to further relieve cord pressure.
- Complete confinement for a minimum of 2 weeks after surgery

NURSING CARE
- Daily physical therapy
- Padded resting surface to decrease the formation of ulcers over pressure points
- Bladder expression or maintenance of an indwelling catheter

INFORMATION FOR CLIENTS
- Treatment of these cases can be costly and often requires referral to a specialist.
- The animal will require extensive nursing care.
- Even in the best of circumstances, some residual neurologic deficit may remain.
- The prognosis for spinal cord trauma will depend on the neurologic examination results. Absence of deep pain for >24 hours has a poor prognosis. Worsening of clinical signs is another indicator of a poor outcome. Recovery time may extend to months in some cases.
- Keep pets confined or on a leash to avoid the possibility of traumatic injury to the spinal cord.

CERVICAL SPINAL CORD DISEASES

ATLANTOAXIAL SUBLUXATION (ATLANTOAXIAL INSTABILITY)

Atlantoaxial subluxation is seen most frequently in young (<1 year) toy and miniature breeds of dogs and occasionally in other breeds. Spinal cord trauma occurs when the cranial portion of the axis is displaced into the spinal column. This displacement may occur as a result of congenital or developmental abnormalities, trauma, or a combination of both.

There is speculation that the mechanism is similar to that of femoral head necrosis (Legg-Calve-Perthes disease) seen in these breeds.

CLINICAL SIGNS
- Reluctance to be patted on the head
- Neck pain
- Presence or absence of tetraparesis or tetraplegia
- Sudden death due to respiratory paralysis

DIAGNOSIS

- Radiographs: Lateral projection with the neck in slight ventriflexion. Care must be taken to avoid further spinal cord damage when positioning the animal. Other congenital abnormalities of the cervical vertebrae may be present.

ⓘ TECH ALERT

Avoid anesthesia if possible when obtaining radiographs of these animals. The decrease in muscle tone during anesthesia may result in further subluxation and spinal cord damage.

TREATMENT

MEDICAL

- Splint neck in extension with strict cage confinement for 6 weeks.
- Treat as for other spinal cord traumas.

SURGICAL

- Stabilization and/or decompression is necessary if the animal has neurologic deficits or neck pain unresponsive to medical treatment.
    1. Dorsal—stainless steel wire is used to attach the dorsal process of the axis to the arch of the atlas. NOTE: Surgery may further damage the cord during positioning and placement of the suture material.
    2. Ventral—bone grafts and cross-pinning technique are accomplished to fuse the axis to the atlas. A neck brace is placed for 2 to 4 weeks postoperatively.
    3. Hemilaminectomy to relieve spinal cord compression.

INFORMATION FOR CLIENTS

- Prognosis is fair to good for animals with mild signs.
- Affected animals should not be used for breeding, because this condition may be hereditary.

CERVICAL SPONDYLOMYELOPATHY (WOBBLER SYNDROME)

Cervical spinal cord compression as a result of caudal vertebral (C5-C7) malformation or misarticulation occurs in large breed dogs, predominantly Great Danes (males) and Doberman Pinschers.

The onset of clinical signs occurs before 1 year of age in the Great Dane and after 2 years of age in the Doberman. Signs are normally progressive and involve hind limb ataxia (a wobbly gait). Pelvic limbs may cross each other, abduct widely, or tend to collapse. The animal may drag its toes, producing abrasions on the dorsal surface or wearing of the nails dorsally. Proprioception will be abnormal. Some animals will have similar lesions in the thoracic limbs. Neurologic examination will be abnormal when testing postural reactions, hopping, and proprioception.

CLINICAL SIGNS
- History of progressive pelvic limb ataxia
- Abnormal wearing of the dorsal surface of the rear paws and/or nails
- Swinging or wobbly gait in the rear limbs
- Gait worse on rising
- Similar signs in front limbs
- Presence or absence of atrophy of scapular muscles
- Rigid flexion of neck without neck pain

DIAGNOSIS
- CBC and serum chemistries should be performed to rule out hypothyroidism or other metabolic defects.
- Radiographs may indicate malalignment or "slipping" of the vertebrae or may indicate remodeling, new bone formation, and narrowing of the spinal canal. Myelography is essential to locate the regions of compression.
- CT and MRI are excellent diagnostic tools if available.

TREATMENT
- Without treatment, the prognosis is poor.

MEDICAL
- Antiinflammatory doses of cortisone
- Neck brace
- Cage confinement

SURGICAL

❶ TECH ALERT
Before undertaking surgery, consider the high potential for morbidity and postsurgical complications.

- Decompression of the spinal cord by laminectomy or ventral slot procedures

- Stabilization of vertebral column:
    Use wire and lag screws dorsally.
    Use ventral approach with spinal fusion and an orthopedic implant to maintain distraction during healing.

INFORMATION FOR CLIENTS
- Overall, the prognosis for these dogs is guarded.
- This is most likely a hereditary defect.
- Dogs with multiple levels of compression have a less favorable prognosis than those with a single level of compression.
- Surgery is risky and costly, and some animals may develop other areas of compression after surgery.

DEGENERATIVE MYELOPATHY

Degenerative myelopathy is a disease seen primarily in the German Shepherd and German Shepherd mixed breed dogs. Other breeds may include Collies, Siberian Huskies, Labrador Retrievers, and Kerry Blue Terriers. There may be a genetic basis for the disease; however, evidence to support a hereditary susceptibility is lacking. Although the exact etiology is unknown, it has been suggested that the disease may result from an autoimmune response to an antigen in the nervous system.

The lesion consists of a diffuse degeneration of white matter in both the ascending and descending tracts in all segments of the spinal cord. The lesion is most extensive in the thoracic region. The affected dog is usually an older animal (>5 years) with a 5- to 6-month history of progressive ataxia and paresis in the rear limbs. Loss of proprioception is often the first indication of a problem. Owners often report that the animal "falls down" when attempting to defecate. There may be muscle wasting from disuse in the caudal thoracic and lumbosacral areas. Symptoms slowly progress until the animal is unable to support weight with the rear limbs.

CLINICAL SIGNS
- Slowly progressive hind limb paresis and ataxia
- Muscle atrophy

DIAGNOSIS
NEUROLOGIC EXAM
- Lesion in the region of T3-L3
- Decreased or absent proprioception and placing reactions

- Increased to normal patellar reflexes
- Lack of pain
- Normal sphincter tone
- Normal panniculus reflex

RADIOGRAPHS

- Radiographs may show dural ossification or narrowed disk spaces but will be normal in most cases.

CEREBROSPINAL FLUID (CSF)

- CSF may show increased protein concentrations from the lumbar subarachnoid space.

TREATMENT

- There is no treatment for this disease. The symptoms will slowly progress until the dog is nonambulatory. Corticosteroids will not improve the symptoms.

INFORMATION FOR CLIENTS

- This is a progressive, incurable disease.
- This disease is not hip dysplasia. It involves a degeneration of the spinal nerves that is irreversible.
- When the dog can no longer support weight, it is time to consider euthanasia.

DISCOSPONDYLITIS (VERTEBRAL OSTEOMYELITIS)

Discospondylitis results when bacteria or fungi become implanted in the bones of the vertebral column. Implantation may occur through hematogenous routes, from penetrating wounds, paravertebral abscess or infection, surgery on the vertebral column, or migrating grass awns. Grass awns are sharp pieces of plant material that migrate through the skin into the spinal bone, causing infection. Discospondylitis is seen in both the cat and the dog, with large and giant breeds being more commonly affected.

Hematogenous spread is probably the most common cause of discospondylitis. Urinary tract infections, bacterial endocarditis, and sites of dental extraction can all be routes for bacterial infection. Organisms typically cultured from lesions include the following: *Brucella canis, Staphylococcus* spp., *Streptococcus canis, Escherichia coli, Corynebacterium* spp., *Proteus* spp., *Pasteurella* spp., *Aspergillus,* and *Mycobacterium.*

Clinical signs of the disease are often nonspecific. If bony proliferation or granulation tissue impinges on the spinal cord, neurologic signs may develop.

CLINICAL SIGNS
- Weight loss

TECH ALERT
Fever of unknown origin

- Depression
- Reluctance to exercise
- Spinal pain
- Hyperesthesia over the lesion(s)
- Presence or absence of neurologic signs

DIAGNOSIS
- Radiographs may show destruction or lysis of bony endplates adjacent to the lesions, osteophyte formation, and collapse of the intervertebral disk space.
- Complete blood count may show elevated WBC.
- CSF may be normal or have elevated protein and WBC.
- Myelography demonstrates areas of spinal compression.
- Aerobic, anaerobic, and fungal cultures of blood, CSF, and urine should be taken.
- *Brucella canis* slide agglutination test should be performed.
- Surgical biopsy and tissue culture are diagnostic.

TREATMENT
- Long-term antibiotic therapy based on culture and sensitivity results or the following:
    Cephalosporins: 30 mg/kg PO q 12 h
    Clindamycin: 11 mg/kg IV, IM, PO q 8 to 12 h
    Enrofloxacin: 15 mg/kg PO q 12 h
    Chloramphenicol: 50 mg/kg PO, IV, IM, SQ, q 8 h
- Continue treatment for at least 6 weeks. It may be necessary to treat for up to 6 months.
- If *Brucella canis* positive:
    Neuter or spay the animal.
    Treat with tetracycline and streptomycin.

ⓘ TECH ALERT

This disease can be transmitted to humans through body fluids. Take care when handling urine and other fluids.

- Provide analgesics for animals exhibiting pain.
- Limit or restrict exercise for the first few weeks of treatment.

INFORMATION FOR CLIENTS

- *Brucella canis* is contagious to humans through urine or in aborted fetal fluids and tissue.
- The prognosis for this disease is guarded.
- Treatment for this disease is costly and long term.
- Periodic reevaluation of radiographs (every 2 to 3 weeks) may be needed to follow treatment response.

ISCHEMIC MYELOPATHY CAUSED BY FIBROCARTILAGINOUS EMBOLISM

This disease most commonly occurs in large and giant breed dogs between the ages of 1 and 9 years. It has been reported in cats and smaller breeds of dogs, but less frequently. Ischemic myelopathy results from necrosis of the spinal cord grey and white fiber tracts when fibrocartilaginous emboli obstruct the veins and arteries in both the leptomeninges and the cord parenchyma. The pathogenesis of the emboli is unknown.

Affected dogs may have a history of mild to moderate exercise before the development of clinical signs. The onset of symptoms is always acute and neurologic deficit may be severe depending on the location of the insult. Symptoms at first may seem progressive but usually stabilize after the first 12 hours. Deficits are usually bilateral and may be asymmetric. A Horner syndrome can be seen if the cervical spine is involved. An embolism in the lumbosacral spinal cord usually produces lower motor neuron signs in the rear limbs, the anal and urinary sphincters, and the tail.

CLINICAL SIGNS

- Large and giant breed dogs are predisposed to this condition.
- Acute onset of neurologic signs
- Lack of acute spinal pain associated with neurologic signs
- Paresis or spastic paralysis of limbs
- Reluctance to move, inability to rise

DIAGNOSIS

- Rule out other causes of myelopathy.
- Radiographs are usually within normal limits.
- CBC is within normal limits.
- CSF is usually within normal limits.
- Myelogram may show mild edema of the cord up to 24 hours after injury.

TREATMENT

- Administer corticosteroids in the same dose as for spinal shock.
- Provide good nursing care to prevent injury to affected structures, limit pressure sores, etc.
- Most animals recover within a few months.

INFORMATION FOR CLIENTS

- The prognosis for this disease is guarded to good.
- Most animals will recover, but it may take months to regain normal function.
- Extensive nursing care may be required to keep the patient comfortable and prevent further injury.

PERIPHERAL NERVOUS SYSTEM

Peripheral nerve disorders are clinically represented by a group of signs known as a *neuropathic syndrome*. The syndrome is commonly associated with trauma to the peripheral, or sometimes the cranial, nerves. Signs of this syndrome include reduced or absent muscle tone, weakness (paresis), or paralysis of the limb or facial muscles followed in 1 to 2 weeks by neurogenic muscular atrophy.

Peripheral neuropathies may involve a single nerve (such as the peroneal, radial, or facial nerve) or multiple nerves (as in polyradiculoneuritis), and the etiology of the neuropathy is often unknown.

DEAFNESS

Deafness in animals may be of central origin, resulting from damage to the central nervous system and auditory pathways, or peripheral, resulting from cochlear abnormalities. Conductive deafness, usually a result of chronic otitis, rupture of the tympanic membrane, or damage to the middle ear, is common in animals.

Neural deafness can be hereditary or congenital, related to drug therapy, or a normal aging change. Deafness seems to be hereditary in Bull Terriers, Dobermans, Rottweilers, pointers, blue-eyed white cats, Dalmatians, Australian Heelers, English Setters, Catahoula, and Australian Shepherds. Animals with congenital deafness suffer from partial or total agenesis of the hearing organ, the organ of Corti, the spiral ganglion, and/or the cochlear nuclei. Drugs that commonly result in ototoxicity include the aminoglycosides (e.g., gentamicin, streptomycin, kanamycin), topical polymyxin B, chloramphenicol, and chlorhexidine with cetrimide.

Hearing impairment is normal in aging pets and is usually related to atrophy of nerve ganglia or cochlear hair cells.

CLINICAL SIGNS
- Lack of response to auditory stimuli
- Excessive sleeping
- A breed prone to deafness

DIAGNOSIS
- Partial loss of hearing and even unilateral complete loss of hearing is difficult to establish on clinical examination of dogs and cats.
- Inability to arouse a sleeping patient with a loud noise (banging a pot, using an air horn, etc.) is diagnostic.
- Behavior evaluation: Stimulate the animal with various sounds from different directions; evaluate the response.
- Physical examination of the external ear canals and the tympanic membrane may assist in reaching a diagnosis.

ELECTRODIAGNOSTIC
- Electrodiagnostic testing usually requires referral to a specialty clinic. Testing may be costly.
- Tympanometry: A probe is inserted into the ear canal and it seals the canal. Sound and pressure changes are delivered through the probe. Tympanic membrane compliance measurements allow the specialist to determine whether the ossicles and/or the tympanic membrane are abnormal.

- Acoustic reflex testing: Delivery of increasing sound pressure levels to the ear evokes the *acoustic reflex* (muscles of the middle ear contract to dampen sound response and prevent damage). If the reflex is present, the auditory system is probably intact.
- Auditory evoked responses: Cochlear function may be assessed by measuring brain electrical responses to either air-conducted clicks from a probe placed in the external ear canal, or from a bone vibrator placed firmly against the mastoid process of the temporal bone. This is especially effective in detecting hereditary and senile deafness. Puppies and kittens should be at least 6 weeks of age for this test to be valid.

TREATMENT
- No treatment is available in most cases. Loss of hearing is permanent.
- Hearing aids are available for animals. Many animals will not tolerate a hearing aid in the ear canal. Because hearing aids are expensive, owners are advised to experiment with foam rubber earplugs in the animal's ear canal before spending money on an actual hearing aid. If the animal will not tolerate the earplugs, it will not tolerate the hearing aid.

INFORMATION FOR CLIENTS
- Hearing loss is permanent. These animals are at risk of injury in their environment, especially in traffic. They may bite when startled.
- If the deafness is hereditary, do not breed the animal.
- Animals can be taught to respond to hand signals rather than voice commands.
- These animals should never be off a leash when outside.
- Keep animals' ears clean and free of infection to avoid damage to the middle and inner ear. It will help to maintain the hearing they have.
- Hearing aids do exist for dogs; however, they are expensive, and many animals will not tolerate them in the ear canal.

Metabolic Neuropathy

Cases of polyneuropathy have been reported in dogs and cats with diabetes mellitus, in dogs with hyperadrenocorticism, and in dogs with hypothyroidism. Clinical signs are variable from progressive weakness to muscle atrophy and depressed spinal reflexes. Paresis and/or paralysis may occur. Hypothyroid dogs show signs related to the cranial nerves, including head tilt, facial paralysis, strabismus, nystagmus, and circling. Good control of the underlying disease is required to limit neurologic damage.

CLINICAL SIGNS

- Varied

DIAGNOSIS

- The underlying disease process can be diagnosed through biochemical testing.
- Rule out other causes of neuropathy.

TREATMENT

- Correct the underlying disease process.

INFORMATION FOR CLIENTS

- The underlying disease process must be controlled with proper medication and frequent reevaluation.
- Treatment for the underlying disease may be lifelong in your pet.

LARYNGEAL PARALYSIS

Hereditary, acquired, and idiopathic laryngeal paralysis occurs in dogs and cats. The hereditary form is seen in the Bouvier des Flandres and in young Siberian Huskies.

Acquired laryngeal paralysis can occur from lead poisoning, rabies, trauma, and inflammatory infiltrates of the vagus nerve. All persons should take care when examining any animal with suspected laryngeal paralysis because rabies is increasing in incidence in many parts of the country.

The idiopathic form has been reported in middle-age to old, large breed and giant breed dogs. Castrated male dogs and cats seem to be more frequently affected than females and nonneutered animals.

CLINICAL SIGNS

- Hereditary: 4 to 6 months of age
- Acquired: 1.5 to 13 years of age
- Inspiratory stridor
- Respiratory distress
- Loss of endurance
- Voice change

- Dyspnea
- Cyanosis
- Complete respiratory collapse

DIAGNOSIS
- Laryngoscopy will reveal laryngeal abductor dysfunction.

TREATMENT
SURGICAL
- Arytenoidectomy
- Arytenoid lateralization
- Removal of the vocal folds

INFORMATION FOR CLIENTS
- The prognosis is guarded to good.
- Do not breed animals that develop hereditary laryngeal paralysis.

MEGAESOPHAGUS

This neurologic disease involves a lack of effective esophageal peristalsis, resulting in dilation of the esophagus and regurgitation of undigested food. The congenital form is common in Great Danes, German Shepherds, Irish Setters, Newfoundlands, Shar-Peis, and Greyhounds. The inherited form is seen in wire-haired Fox Terriers and Miniature Schnauzers.

The congenital form usually becomes evident around weaning time when puppies begin eating solid foods. Chronic regurgitation of undigested food, weight loss, respiratory signs, and pneumonias are seen clinically.

Acquired megaesophagus may occur in animals of any age. The appearance of symptoms may be linked to a variety of causes, such as metabolic neuromuscular disease, distemper, tick paralysis, lead poisoning, laryngeal paralysis–polyneuropathy complex, and polymyositis.

The prognosis for megaesophagus is guarded to poor. Management techniques such as elevated feeding of high caloric diets seem to decrease clinical signs. Feeding regimens vary. It has been suggested that liquid diets be used exclusively (easier for food to enter the stomach by gravity flow) whereas other studies recommend small meatballs of canned food to stimulate what little peristalsis there is. The goal of management is to decrease the frequency of regurgitation, prevent overdistension of the esophagus, and to provide adequate nutrition for the patient.

Several small meals should be fed during the day. Gastrostomy tubes can be placed long term if solid meals are not well tolerated by the patient.

CLINICAL SIGNS
- Regurgitation of undigested food
- Respiratory signs: Cough, dyspnea, drooling, pneumonia
- Lack of growth or weight loss

DIAGNOSIS
- Radiographic evidence of a dilated esophagus to the level of the diaphragm:
  Barium meal—mix barium with canned food. Feed mixture and radiograph.
  Fluoroscopy with a barium swallow.

ⓘ TECH ALERT
Animals with a dilated esophagus full of barium are at risk of aspiration pneumonia. Keep animal in a vertical position for 5 to 10 minutes after the procedure.

- Rule out metabolic causes with serum chemistries, complete physical exam, CBC, etc.

TREATMENT
- Provide elevated feeding platform.
- Provide liquid or soft diet high in caloric density.
- Give several small feedings daily.
- Treat any underlying metabolic disorders.

INFORMATION FOR CLIENTS
- The prognosis for this disease is guarded to poor.
- Treatment aims to decrease clinical signs and prevent the development of aspiration pneumonia. There is no cure.

TICK PARALYSIS

In the United States, the common dog tick *Dermacentor variabilis* and the Rocky Mountain wood tick *Dermacentor andersoni* are most often involved with a flaccid, afebrile, ascending motor paralysis. Cats seem to be resistant to tick paralysis.

The female tick produces a salivary neurotoxin that interferes with acetylcholine concentrations at the neuromuscular junction.

The onset of clinical signs is gradual, beginning as incoordination in the pelvic limbs. Altered voice and dysphasia may be seen. Within 24 to 72 hours, dogs become recumbent. Reflexes are lost while sensation remains. Death may occur owing to respiratory paralysis.

Recovery usually occurs within 1 to 3 days following removal of all ticks on the animal. Animals with respiratory involvement may need to be ventilated until signs subside.

CLINICAL SIGNS
- Gradual development of hind limb incoordination that progresses to a flaccid ascending paralysis
- The presence of ticks on the dog

DIAGNOSIS
- Rule out other causes of neuromuscular disease.

TREATMENT
- Remove *all* ticks from the animal (manually or with a dip).
- Oral cythioate (Proban) can be used to remove hidden ticks (3.3 to 6.6 mg/kg PO).
- Supportive care is required.

COONHOUND PARALYSIS (CHP)/POLYRADICULONEURITIS

CHP has generated intense interest because of its resemblance to Guillain-Barré syndrome in humans. Like the human syndrome, CHP may have an immunologic pathogenesis. However, the exact agent has not yet been isolated. Many, but not all, cases of CHP involve a raccoon bite before the development of clinical signs. Recent reports indicate raccoon saliva contains the etiologic factor for CHP and that only certain susceptible dogs are at risk of developing CHP.

Pathologic findings include segmental demyelination along with degeneration of myelin and axons, especially in the ventral nerve roots.

The disease can affect adult dogs of any breed and either sex. Clinical signs usually appear within 7 to 14 days after exposure to the raccoon, although some dogs develop the disease without exposure to a raccoon bite. Weakness begins in the hind limbs with paralysis progressing rapidly to a flaccid, systemic tetraplegia. Some dogs may be more severely affected. In severely affected animals, there may be an absence of spinal reflexes, loss of voice, labored breathing, and an inability to lift the head. These animals may die from respiratory paralysis. Paralysis may last 2 to 3 months, but the prognosis is generally good for most cases.

CLINICAL SIGNS
- Recent exposure to a raccoon or other nonspecific antigen stimulation
- Ascending, flaccid paralysis
- Alert, afebrile animal

DIAGNOSIS
- Clinical signs (lower motor neuron)
- History of some antigenic stimulation
- Rule out all other metabolic or infectious causes

TREATMENT
- Treatment consists of supportive nursing care.
- Corticosteroids in antiinflammatory doses have been used clinically.
- Support respirations if necessary.

INFORMATION FOR CLIENTS
- Animals can develop this condition without exposure to raccoons.
- Affected animals may require long-term nursing care.
- Some animals may regain total function whereas severely affected animals may not.

FACIAL NERVE PARALYSIS

Idiopathic, acute facial nerve paralysis has been reported in adult dogs and cats (>5 years). The cause of this condition is unknown. Cocker Spaniels, Pembroke Welsh Corgis, Boxers, English Setters, and domestic longhaired cats seem predisposed.

Biopsies of affected facial nerves reveal degeneration of myelinated fibers. The prognosis for complete recovery is guarded.

CLINICAL SIGNS
- Ear droop
- Lip paralysis

- Sialosis
- Deviation of the nose
- Collection of food in the paralyzed side of the mouth
- Absence of menace and palpebral reflex

DIAGNOSIS

- Electrodiagnostic testing of facial nerves
- Clinical signs of acute facial paralysis without signs of trauma

TREATMENT

- Corticosteroids can be provided; however, efficacy is unknown.
- Artificial tears to affected eye help prevent corneal dryness.
- Keep the oral cavity clear of food.

INFORMATION FOR CLIENTS

- The cause of this condition is unknown.
- Complete recovery does not usually occur.
- Animals may develop keratoconjunctivitis sicca owing to damage to the nerves that pass to the lacrimal gland.
- Affected animals may require lifelong maintenance care.

PANSYSTEMIC DISEASES ten

Pansystemic diseases include those that involve multiple body systems in addition to the primary target organ. The etiologies of these diseases may be viral, bacterial, or parasitic, and secondary infections are common. Box 10-1 lists some of the most commonly seen pansystemic diseases of the dog and cat.

FELINE PANLEUKOPENIA (FELINE DISTEMPER)

Feline panleukopenia is caused by a DNA virus of the family Parvoviridae, which is closely related antigenically to the canine parvovirus, type 2. The disease is primarily one of young, unvaccinated cats and feral animals. Transmission is by direct contact or from a contaminated environment. The virus shed into the environment may remain infectious for years.

Feline parvovirus multiplies within mitotic cells of the neonatal brain, bone marrow, lymphoid tissue, and in the intestinal lymphoid tissue, resulting in destruction of the cells with release of a large number of virions. The incubation period is usually 4 to 5 days. Signs may be peracute, acute, subacute, or subclinical.

CLINICAL SIGNS
- Fever
- Depression
- Vomiting
- Fetid diarrhea
- Dehydration
- Anorexia
- Fetal death, abortion, or reabsorption in the pregnant queen
- Cerebellar or retinal defects in neonates

Box 10-1.   Common pansystemic diseases

FELINE
- Feline leukemia
- Feline immunodeficiency virus
- Feline infectious peritonitis
- Feline panleukopenia
- Toxoplasmosis

CANINE
- Canine distemper
- Canine rabies
- Canine parvovirus
- Ehrlichiosis
- Lyme disease

DIAGNOSIS
- Complete blood count: Moderate to severe panleukopenia
- Positive fecal test using CITE test for canine parvovirus
- Serum antibody titers
- Viral isolation

TREATMENT

 TECH ALERT
Isolate these cats from other animals. All body secretions contain virus.

AGGRESSIVE SUPPORTIVE THERAPY
- Maintain hydration and electrolyte balance.
- Force feed after vomiting is controlled.
- Broad-spectrum antibiotics are required.

INFORMATION FOR CLIENTS
- Cats who survive the infection develop a lifelong immunity.
- To prevent disease, kittens should be vaccinated between 8 and 10 weeks of age, then again after 12 to 14 weeks. Yearly boosters should be given to all cats. (New vaccination guidelines may be available in the near future.)

FELINE INFECTIOUS PERITONITIS (FIP)

Feline infectious peritonitis (FIP) is primarily a disease of catteries and multi-cat households. FIP does not occur without exposure to feline coronavirus. Eighty percent to 90% of cats in catteries have antibodies to feline coronaviruses (mostly feline enteric coronavirus [FECV]), and these cats shed virus intermittently. FECV is highly contagious through the feces as well as urine and saliva. Current thinking is that this virus may mutate to FIPV within some infected cats. FIPV then enters the macrophages, spreading throughout the body.

FIPV and FECV are difficult to differentiate with current testing procedures. Enzyme-linked immunosorbent assay (ELISA) and immunofluorescence assays are nonspecific for FIPV. Even the polymerase chain reaction (PCR) cannot differentiate the two viruses.

FIP occurs in two forms: the effusive, or "wet," form (75%) and the noneffusive, or "dry," form. About 45% of cats having the dry form will have ocular or neurologic lesions. In the effusive form, perivasculitis results in the accumulation of a protein-rich fluid in the thoracic and/or abdominal cavity, the scrotum, the pericardial cavity, and the renal subcapsular space. The inflammatory process may also involve the liver and the pancreas. The clinical progression is more rapid than with the dry form.

Signs of noneffusive FIP are more vague. The pyogranulomatous lesions may be found anywhere in the body, especially the eyes and the neurologic system. Clinical signs may include ataxia, seizures, behavorial changes, paresis, and/or hyperesthesia. Ocular signs include iritis, retinitis, uveitis, hyphema, corneal edema, retinal hemorrhage, and retinal detachment.

CLINICAL SIGNS
WET FORM
- Ascites, pleural effusion
- Anorexia
- Depression
- Weight loss
- Dehydration
- May or may not be febrile

DRY FORM
- Fever of unknown origin
- Anorexia

- Depression
- Weight loss
- Ocular lesions
- Neurologic signs
- Enlarged kidneys (uncommon)

DIAGNOSIS
- Clinical signs
- Rule out other diseases.
- Cytology and chemical analysis of abdominal and pleural fluid show the following:
    Viscous, clear to yellow fluid
    <20,000 nucleated cells/μl
    Protein-rich (>3.5 g/dl)
    Albumin/globulin ratio <0.81
- High antibody titers may be *suggestive* of FIP.

TREATMENT
SUPPORTIVE
- Aspirate pleural/abdominal fluids to make cat more comfortable.
- Steroids (prednisolone 2.2 to 4.4 mg/kg daily)
- Broad-spectrum antibiotics

IMMUNOTHERAPY
- ImmunoRegulin
- Ribavirin and adenine arabinoside inhibit FIPV in cell culture (clinical effect unknown).

PREVENTION
- Isolate pregnant queens 2 weeks before giving birth.
- Remove weaning kittens from queens by 5 weeks of age.
- Vaccinate seronegative cats with Primucell FIP (Pfizer), an intranasal vaccine, at 16 weeks of age. This drug provides good protection against FIP but is not effective in cats already exposed to FECV.

INFORMATION FOR CLIENTS
- The virus is inactivated in the environment by most household disinfectants.

- Diagnosis of this disease can be difficult and may require a series of expensive tests to rule out other possibilities.

FELINE LEUKEMIA VIRUS (FeLV)

Feline leukemia is caused by a coronavirus that is associated with both neoplastic and nonneoplastic (immunosuppressive) disease. Both vertical and horizontal transmission occurs. The virus is very unstable in the environment; therefore close contact between cats is required for infection to occur. The virus can be isolated from saliva, urine, tears, and milk and can be spread through fighting, grooming, or exposure to contaminated food bowls, food, water, or litter pans. Transplacental and transmammary transmission does occur. The outcome of exposure to the virus is variable and depends on several host factors: age, immunocompetence, concurrent disease, viral strain, dose, and the duration of exposure.

Exposed cats may (1) develop a regressive infection (transient), (2) develop a progressive infection (persistent viremia) with no clinical signs, or (3) develop active infection with clinical signs. Clinical signs associated with FeLV include anemia, anorexia, depression, weight loss, nervous system disease, and secondary infections. Vomiting and diarrhea may be seen if the gastrointestinal tract is involved.

Lymphoma is the most common FeLV-associated neoplastic disease. Tumors can occur in the thymus, the alimentary tract, or in various lymph nodes throughout the body.

Treatment is primarily supportive, and prevention is through vaccination and limited contact with infected cats. All cats should be tested for feline leukemia using the standard peripheral-blood ELISA test before vaccination. If positive, cats should undergo an IFA test or be retested by ELISA in 3 to 4 months. Cats remaining positive will usually be positive for life and should be isolated from all other nonvaccinated cats. Many may remain in good health for prolonged periods if not stressed.

CLINICAL SIGNS
- Fever
- Anorexia
- Weight loss
- Anemia

- Secondary infections
- Vomiting and diarrhea
- Abortion
- Renal disease
- Tumors of lymphoid origin
- Neurologic signs

DIAGNOSIS

- Feline leukemia positive on ELISA test
- Complete blood count: Nonregenerative anemia
- IFA positive
- Clinical signs of recurring infections

TREATMENT

HUSBANDRY

- FeLV-positive cats should be isolated from all other cats.
- FeLV-positive cats should be kept indoors.
- FeLV-positive cats should be vaccinated for other feline diseases and rabies on a routine schedule.
- Eliminate stress in affected cats.

MEDICAL (THERE IS NO CURE)

- Immunomodulator drugs:
    Acemannan (CarringtonLab): 100 mg/cat PO, SQ daily or 2 mg/kg IP once a week for 6 weeks
    Propionibacterium acnes (ImmunoRegulin): 0.5 ml/cat IV 1 to 2 times weekly
    Human recombinant interferon-α (r-HuIFN-α; Roferon, Roche): 30 U q 24 h PO for 7 days, repeated every other week
- Antiviral drugs:
    AZT: 15 mg/kg PO q 12 h
    9-(2-phosphomethoxyethyl) adenine (PMEA): 2.5 mg/kg SQ q 12 h

---

❶ TECH ALERT

These drugs are toxic to bone marrow. Cats should have hemograms reevaluated frequently during treatment. Limit treatment to 3-week course to avoid marrow toxicity.

- Broad-spectrum antibiotics to control secondary infections
- Appetite stimulants:
    Oxazepam (Serax, Wyeth): 2.5 mg/kg PO
    Diazepam (Valium, Roche): 0.2 mg/kg IV
- Chemotherapy for solid tumors

INFORMATION FOR CLIENTS
- A healthy FeLV-positive cat need not be euthanized.
- If your cat is positive for FeLV you should do the following:
    Keep the animal indoors.
    Isolate from all other cats.
    Keep up with vaccinations.
    See your veterinarian if any signs of disease develop.

ⓘ TECH ALERT
The public health significance of FeLV is controversial. The virus does grow in human cell cultures, although there is no evidence of the infection in any nonfeline species. *However,* immunosuppressed humans, pregnant women, and neonates should not be exposed to FeLV-positive cats.

FELINE IMMUNODEFICIENCY VIRUS (FIV OR FELINE AIDS)

Feline immunodeficiency virus is a lentivirus associated with an immunodeficiency disease in domestic cats, which is morphologically and biochemically similar to the HIV virus but is antigenically distinct. FIV is highly species specific, growing only in feline-derived cells. Most infections are acquired by horizontal transmission among adult cats. Male, sexually intact cats living outdoors are at greatest risk of developing FIV infection. Fighting and bite wounds seem to be the major route of transmission. There is little or no sexual transmission in cats. Neonatal kittens may become infected by contact with infected queens, although plasma antibodies against FIV may be passed to kittens in colostrum when nursing. Because the ELISA test for FIV detects antibodies, kittens should not be diagnosed using these tests until after 6 months of age.

Clinical signs of FIV involve chronic, unresponsive infections (gingivitis, stomatitis, and skin, ear, and/or respiratory tract infections), anemia, ocular and/or neurologic signs, and weight loss. Chronic fever and cachexia are common findings. Cats may remain symptom-free for long periods after infection or may suffer from recurring bouts of illness interspersed with periods of relatively good health. Cats infected with FIV are at increased risk for development of chronic renal insufficiency.

There is no vaccine available at the present time. Prevention of infection is by limiting exposure to outdoor cats. Spaying and neutering outdoor cats can limit exposure by decreasing aggressive behaviors.

CLINICAL SIGNS
- History of recurrent bouts of illnesses
- Cachexia, anorexia
- Gingivitis, stomatitis
- Chronic, nonresponsive ear or skin infections
- Chronic upper respiratory infections
- Diarrhea
- Vomiting
- Neurologic disorders
- Ocular disease (anterior uveitis, glaucoma)
- Pale mucous membranes
- Chronic fever

DIAGNOSIS
- Clinical history
- Positive ELISA test (blood)
- Complete blood count: Anemia, lymphopenia

TREATMENT
HUSBANDRY
- Keep infected cats indoors.
- Isolate if aggressive to other cats in the household.
- Transmission from fomites or casual contact is unlikely.

MEDICAL (NO CURE FOR DISEASE)
- Immunomodulator drugs:
    Acemannan (Carrington Labs): 100 mg/cat PO, SQ daily or 2 mg/kg IP weekly for 6 weeks
    ImmunoRegulin (Immunovet): 0.5 ml/cat IV 1 to 2 times weekly

Interferon-α (Intron-A, Schering-Plough): 0.5 to 30 U/cat PO q 24 h for 5 days on alternate weeks

- Antiviral therapy: AZT (Retrovir, Glaxo-Wellcome): 15 mg/kg PO q 12 h. If anemia develops, stop medication until CBC returns to normal then restart at previous dose and increase to original dose over 1 to 2 weeks.

SURGICAL

- Whole mouth extraction of teeth may be necessary in cats with chronic stomatitis and gingivitis.

INFORMATION FOR CLIENTS

- FIV poses *no* health hazard for humans.
- Infected cats may survive for prolonged periods of time before developing advanced stages of the disease.
- For cats with severe gingivitis and stomatitis, tooth extraction may be the best course of treatment. Cats are able to eat well even after whole mouth extractions.
- Keeping your pet indoors will prevent infection.
- Keeping an infected cat free from stress and concurrent disease is *extremely* important.

TOXOPLASMOSIS

Toxoplasmosis is caused by *Toxoplasma gondii,* an intracellular coccidian parasite with worldwide distribution. The feline is the only definitive host, but other warm-blooded animals, including man, can serve as intermediate hosts. Exposure to *Toxoplasma* is common; an estimated 30% to 60% of adult humans are seropositive for exposure.

Transmission can occur by three routes: (1) eating contaminated meat from an intermediate host, (2) fecal-oral route, and (3) transplacental route. In carnivores, ingestion of infected intermediate hosts is responsible for most infections.

Once sporulated oocysts are ingested, tachyzoites form and invade any tissue in the body. Clinical signs of disease are related to the tissue involved. The disease may be especially severe in immunocompromised animals or in very young animals. In the cat, the two tissues most commonly involved are the lung and the eyes, whereas in the dog, the gastrointestinal, neurologic, and the respiratory systems are commonly infected. However, *Toxoplasma* infections are rare in the dog.

After infection, the cat sheds oocysts in the feces for 1 to 2 weeks. Because of this limited shedding of organisms, exposure to these infective oocysts is probably not an important source of infection for humans and other cats. Ingestion of uncooked or undercooked meat is most likely the main route of infection in both cats and humans. Therefore, prevention of infection involves eliminating hunting and feeding of raw meat to the cat, cooking all meat properly before feeding, and following good hygiene practices when handling cat feces.

Humans who are immunosuppressed should avoid contact with infected cats. Congenital infection in the first or second trimester can result in serious birth defects. Although infected cats are unlikely to pose a major threat to most pregnant women, there are some steps that can be taken to prevent infection:

- Avoid feeding raw meat to cats.
- Keep cats indoors.
- Have someone else clean the litter box daily. Rinse litter box weekly with hot water.
- Avoid the use of immunosuppressive drugs in the seropositive cat.
- Have yourself checked for antibody before becoming pregnant.
- Avoid acquiring a new cat during pregnancy.
- Wash hands thoroughly and wear gloves when gardening.
- Cook all meat properly.
- *Do not panic*. Speak with your doctor and veterinarian when you determine you are pregnant. You should not have to get rid of your pets.

CLINICAL SIGNS
Signs will depend on the organs involved.

- Anorexia
- Lethargy
- Fever
- Weight loss
- Diarrhea
- Vomiting
- Icterus
- Respiratory disease
- Lameness
- Pancreatic disease
- Anterior uveitis
- Glaucoma

- CNS disease
- Sudden death

DIAGNOSIS

> **① TECH ALERT**
>
> **Antemortem diagnosis is difficult because of the presence of antibodies found in the general population and the lack of long-term shedding of oocysts in the infected cat.**

- Complete blood count: Nonspecific, variable changes
- Serum chemistries:
    Increases in ALT, ALP, and total bilirubin may occur.
    Creatine kinase is often elevated.
- Thoracic radiographs may show diffuse lesions with or without pleural effusion.
- ELISA test should be available to test for *Toxoplasma* sp.–specific IgG, IgM, and antigen-containing immune complexes.
- Paired titers having a fourfold increase are required for a presumptive diagnosis (IgM >1 : 256 and increased IgG).

TREATMENT
- Clindamycin is the drug of choice for treatment: 25 mg/kg PO, IM divided into 2 doses daily for 2 to 3 weeks.

INFORMATION FOR CLIENTS
- See section above outlining advice to pregnant women. *Do not panic.*

RABIES (FELINE AND CANINE)

Although rabies technically is not a pansystemic disease, it has been placed in this chapter because exposure of veterinary technicians and veterinarians often occurs during the examination of animals with vague and seemingly unrelated symptoms. Examples include the cat or dog with hypersalivation (which could indicate dental disease, foreign body), the pet with rear leg paralysis (possible trauma, tick paralysis, disc disease), and the wild or exotic pet that is listless or "just not doing right." People often have no idea that their pet or the animal they have just rescued from the woods may be infected with the rabies virus.

Rabies is a viral-induced neurologic disease of warm-blooded animals. It has a worldwide distribution. In the United States, raccoons, bats, skunks, foxes, and coyotes serve as the major wild animal hosts for the disease. The virus is spread through the saliva of the infected animal and may enter the body through a bite, open wound, or mucous membranes. Aerosol transmission has been documented. The incubation time from exposure to the onset of clinical disease is usually 3 to 8 weeks, but in some cases it may be longer. During this time the virus enters the nerve endings around the bite or wound and ascends the nerve to the brain where it multiplies in the neurons. It then travels along nerves to the salivary glands where it appears in the saliva.

Rabies is characterized by three stages: (1) the prodromal stage, (2) the excitative (furious) stage, and (3) the paralytic stage. The prodromal stage is characterized by changes in behavior (wild animals become friendly, nocturnal animals come out during the day, dogs and cats become fearful or apprehensive), and it is during this stage that people are at the greatest risk of exposure. During the excitative phase, the animal may appear hyperreactive. They may attack unprovoked or attack inanimate objects. Some may appear to be in a stupor ("dumb" rabies). The first two stages are followed by the paralytic stage in which the animal experiences an ascending paralysis of the hind limb eventually leading to respiratory paralysis and death. These three stages may be completed in less than 1 week.

The technician should be alert to the early symptoms of rabies to prevent accidental exposure. Always get a vaccination history and wear gloves when examining the oral cavity of an animal. Avoid handling wildlife brought in by clients, and take precautions with domestically raised skunks and raccoons. Rabies has no cure and is almost always a fatal disease. Protect yourself from exposure by following these guidelines:
- Obtain preexposure prophylaxis (vaccines are available).
- Wear gloves when examining any animal's oral cavity and during necropsy procedures.
- Promote vaccination of all dogs, cats, and horses.
- Advise clients to leave wildlife in the wild.
- Assume rabies is a possibility in all animals presenting with neurologic symptoms or voice changes.

CLINICAL SIGNS
- Behavioral changes
- Difficulty swallowing
- Hypersalivation

- Extruded penis
- Hind limb ataxia
- Depression, stupor

DIAGNOSIS
- Postmortem examination of brain tissue is definitive.
- Positive FA test for virus in the brain and brainstem. No antemortem test is available.

TREATMENT
- None. If suspected, the animal should be euthanized. Exposed staff should receive postexposure treatment. Vaccinated animals exposed to a rabid animal should be revaccinated and observed for 90 days. Unvaccinated animals exposed to rabies should be euthanized or kept under *strict* isolation for 6 months. Rules for quarantine may vary with location.

INFORMATION FOR CLIENTS
- Well-vaccinated pets create a buffer zone against human infection.
- Never handle wild animals that appear tame or friendly.
- Avoid promoting visitations by raccoons and skunks by covering garbage cans and not leaving food out for them.
- Diagnosis requires intact brain tissue. Avoid injuring the brain when euthanizing the animal.
- If your pet bites a person, it must be quarantined for 10 days at your expense. This quarantine may be at a veterinary clinic or humane shelter. Animals showing no signs of disease after 10 days are considered to have been uninfected at the time of the bite. *The quarantine is to protect humans, not your pet.*

CANINE DISTEMPER

Canine viral distemper (CVD) is a highly contagious viral disease of dogs and other carnivores. The incidence of disease is highest in dogs 3 to 6 months of age. Canine distemper virus is a paramyxovirus that is relatively labile in the environment. Most routine cleaning agents, disinfectants, and heat will readily destroy the virus.

CVD is transmitted through aerosolization of body secretions. There are several strains of the virus that vary in virulence from mild to fatal. The hallmark of infection is immunosuppression followed by the development of secondary infections. Clinical signs usually associated with distemper are related to the presence of the secondary infections, although encephalitis and other neurologic signs may be due to the direct effect of the virus on neurons.

A diagnosis of distemper is usually based on clinical signs in an unvaccinated animal but FA testing is available. The only treatment is supportive. The fatality rate may be as high as 90% depending on the strain involved. A good vaccination program is the best prevention.

CLINICAL SIGNS
- Fever
- Cough
- Mucopurulent nasal and ocular discharge
- Pneumonia
- Anorexia
- Vomiting
- Diarrhea
- Dehydration
- Abdominal pustules
- Hyperkeratosis of foot pads
- "Chewing gum" seizures (clonus)
- Muscle twitching
- Ataxia, circling, blindness

DIAGNOSIS
- Physical exam and history
- Serology: Rising titers in paired serum samples
- Fluorescent antibody test to detect the virus in epithelial cells collected from the conjunctiva or other mucous membranes

TREATMENT
- Antibiotics, fluids, nutrition, and vitamins are supportive measures.
- There is no specific treatment for the virus.
- There is no specific treatment for clonus.

INFORMATION FOR CLIENTS
- A good vaccination program for all dogs is the only prevention.
- The prognosis is guarded especially if neurologic signs are present.

- CDV is the most common cause of seizures in dogs less than 6 months of age.
- Neurologic signs may appear weeks to years after the actual infection with CDV.

CANINE PARVOVIRUS

Canine parvovirus is a common cause of infectious enteritis in the dog. The disease is caused by a single-stranded, nonenveloped DNA virus and is closely related to the virus that causes feline panleukopenia. The virus is one of the most resistant viruses known, often surviving for years in contaminated environments. The virus was first isolated in 1978 and was associated with an outbreak of hemorrhagic gastroenteritis with a high mortality. Parvovirus is primarily a disease of young puppies lacking sufficient antibody protection. The virus is spread via feces and transmission is by the fecal-oral route. The virus invades rapidly dividing cells of the lymphoid system, the intestinal tract, the bone marrow, and the myocardium (in utero or shortly after birth). Factors such as age, stress, genetics, and concurrent intestinal parasitism influence the severity of the disease. Dobermans and Rottweilers have a higher likelihood of severe disease than most other breeds.

Animals infected with parvovirus may become febrile and lethargic followed several days later by anorexia, depression, vomiting, and bloody, foul-smelling diarrhea. These animals quickly become dehydrated. Viral invasion of the bone marrow and lymph system produces a profound lymphopenia and neutropenia in severely infected dogs (WBC may be <2000). Puppies can become hypoglycemic and hypokalemic from lack of nutritional intake. Secondary sepsis may occur along with possible intestinal intussusceptions.

Diagnosis is by fecal ELISA test for the parvo antigen (CITE, IDEXX). Treatment consists of aggressive supportive therapy including IV fluids, antibiotics, antiemetics, antiinflammatories, and colony stimulating factor (Nupogen, Amgen). Vaccination is the best preventive measure. Clients should avoid exposing their pets to other animals until their pets have established firm immunity (usually between 18 and 22 weeks of age, before the last parvo booster is given). Yearly boosters are recommended for most animals. In high-risk breeds, a booster every 6 months may be required.

CLINICAL SIGNS

- Young puppy or older, unvaccinated dog

TECH ALERT

The disease has been seen in older vaccinated animals and in animals whose owners purchased vaccines from livestock stores or through catalogues.

- Depression
- Lethargy
- Anorexia
- Vomiting
- Bloody diarrhea
- Dehydration
- Fever

DIAGNOSIS

- Positive fecal ELISA test
- CBC: Marked lymphopenia and neutropenia—increased packed cell volume (PCV)
- Serum chemistries (not specific for CPV):
    Hypoglycemia
    Hyponatremia
    Metabolic acidosis
    Hypokalemia
- Fecal examination to rule out intestinal parasites
- Serology: High titer (1 : 10,000) for CPV

TREATMENT

TECH ALERT

These animals are highly infectious and should be handled in isolation.

SUPPORTIVE

- IV fluids: Crystalloids are the fluids of choice
- Potassium chloride added: 8 mEq/500 ml of fluid
- Dextrose added as needed: 5% solution

❶ TECH ALERT

Avoid SQ fluids because these animals are prone to infections from repeated injections through the skin. Also, maintain good asepsis of catheter sites, changing catheters every 48 to 72 hours if possible. Keep bandages dry and clean.

- Antibiotics:
  Ampicillin: 10 to 40 mg/kg IV, SQ q 6 to 8 h
  Amikacin: 5 to 10 mg/kg IV, SQ q 8 h
  Gentamicin: 2 to 4 mg/kg IV, SQ q 6 to 8 h

❶ TECH ALERT

Avoid fluoroquinolones in young animals because they damage cartilage.

- Antiemetics:
  Reglan: 0.2 to 0.5 mg/kg IV, SQ q 6 to 8 h
  Flunixin meglumine: 0.25 mg/kg IV, SQ, or IM; may repeat in 12 to 24 hours (for pyrexia)
- Colony-stimulating factors: Promote maturation and release of specific cells from bone marrow (may not be of value)
  RhG-CSF/filgastrim (Nupogen, Amgen): 5 µg/kg SQ q 24 h
- Nutrition: Partial parenteral nutrition until the patient goes 24 hours without vomiting

PREVENTION
- Vaccinate puppies beginning at 6 to 8 weeks of age with boosters every 3 to 4 weeks until 16 weeks of age. Revaccinate high-risk breeds at 22 weeks of age. Rebooster all dogs yearly. (Fecal parvo antigen tests may be weakly positive for 5 to 15 days after vaccination.)

INFORMATION FOR CLIENTS
- Make sure you have your new puppy vaccinated on a proper schedule. See your veterinarian.
- Many puppies can survive parvovirus infection with proper treatment. Some clinics report 80% to 90% success rates.
- Treatment may be expensive and require a hospital stay of several weeks.

- Other dogs in the house may become infected if not adequately vaccinated.
- The virus can survive long term in the environment.
- Keep puppies free of intestinal parasites. Intestinal parasites seem to predispose dogs to parvovirus infection.

⚠ TECH ALERT

Tips for technicians dealing with parvovirus:
- Isolate all patients suspected of parvovirus infection until a diagnosis is confirmed. These patients should not be seen in the exam area used for well-patient exams. Take animals suspected of infection directly to the isolation ward.
- All waste and bedding should be disposed of directly from the isolation area.
- Wear protective clothing and shoe covers when treating these patients in isolation. Do not wear these clothes into the rest of the clinic.
- Affected animals require intensive care to keep clean and dry. Frequent vomiting and bloody diarrhea are unpleasant for the staff but must not be allowed to accumulate. Secondary infections to wet skin and catheter sites can develop if patients are not cleaned frequently.
- Do not allow these puppies to become overhydrated. Carefully monitor fluid intake.

RICKETTSIOSES

Rickettsiae are small, gram-negative, obligate, intracellular bacterial organisms. Of the three known families, two—*Rickettsiae* and *Ehrlichieae*—are pathogens of dogs. Both of these organisms are tick-borne pathogens, with infection occurring through the saliva during feeding by the tick. Distribution and seasonal occurrence of these diseases are related to the life cycle of the corresponding tick. Transmission of the organism requires attachment of the tick to the host for 5 to 20 hours.

ROCKY MOUNTAIN SPOTTED FEVER

The causative agent of this disease, *Rickettsia rickettsii,* induces vascular endothelial injury. The disease is spread by the ticks *Dermacentor variabilis* and *Dermacentor andersoni*. The transmitted rickettsiae replicate in vascular endothelial cells, resulting in inflammation, necrosis, and increased vascular permeability. Clinical signs are related to the areas of inflammation. Pulmonary, CNS, myocardial, ocular, renal, and musculoskeletal systems may be involved.

Clinical signs of edema, hypotension, shock, conduction abnormalities, heart blocks or arrhythmia, seizures, coma, pulmonary edema, retinal hemorrhages, and acute renal failure may be seen in infected dogs. These signs are vague and may mimic other infectious and noninfectious diseases. Diagnosis requires a direct immunofluorescent test for *R. rickettsii* in skin or tissue biopsy.

Tetracycline or doxycycline are the treatments of choice; rapid improvement is seen after initiation of therapy. Owners should be educated as to the risk of tick exposure and the possibility of human infection through the environment.

CLINICAL SIGNS
- Fever
- Anorexia
- Depression
- Mucopurulent ocular discharge
- Tachypnea
- Coughing
- Vomiting and diarrhea
- Muscle pain
- CNS signs
- Severe weight loss
- Retinal hemorrhages
- Scrotal edema

❶ TECH ALERT
This disease usually appears in the spring and summer months.

DIAGNOSIS
- Direct immunofluorescent test of tissue biopsy
- Indirect immunofluorescent test showing a fourfold increase in serum titers
- History of tick exposure
- Complete blood count:
    Anemia
    Leukopenia to leukocytosis
    Thrombocytopenia

- Serum chemistry:
    Increased ALT
    Increased ALP
    Hypoproteinemia
    Hypocalcemia
    Hyponatremia

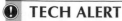

TECH ALERT

Blood from these patients may be infectious to persons handling it. Avoid contact by wearing protective clothing. Avoid blood from the tick as well.

TREATMENT

- Tetracycline: 22 mg/kg t.i.d. q 14 days
- Doxycycline: 10 mg/kg q 14 days
- Monitor fluid intake carefully to avoid exacerbation of the edema already present.

INFORMATION FOR CLIENTS

- If you develop signs of an upper respiratory tract infection, fever, headache, myalgia, or abdominal pain, see your doctor.
- Supportive care is very important for infected animals and should be performed under careful veterinary supervision.
- Antibiotics only reduce the number of organisms; the animal must have a good immune response to eliminate them.
- Control of tick infestation is the best way to prevent the disease. Keep pets out of heavily infested areas, and remove ticks quickly.

CANINE MONOCYTIC EHRLICHIOSIS

This rickettsial disease is caused by *Ehrlichia canis,* whose vector tick is *Rhipicephalus sanguineus,* the brown dog tick. Although diagnosed primarily in the southeastern and southwestern United States, the disease first gained attention as a devastating disease of military working dogs in Vietnam. Following infection, *E. canis* causes acute, subclinical, and chronic disease phases. The acute stage lasts between 2 and 4 weeks, during which time the organism multiplies within circulating mononuclear cells and cells of the spleen and liver. Infected mononuclear cells are transported to other organs such as the lungs, kidneys, and meninges. A resulting vasculitis and subendothelial tissue infection develops. The subclinical phase appears 6 to 9 weeks after infection.

Dogs may not show clinical signs during this period before progressing to the chronic phase. During the chronic phase, bone marrow is suppressed, resulting in thrombocytopenia, nonregenerative anemia, and pancytopenia. Some dogs with chronic disease will develop glomerulonephritis.

Diagnosis is by indirect immunofluorescent antibody technique. Tetracycline or doxycycline is the treatment of choice, and the prognosis is generally good.

CLINICAL SIGNS
ACUTE PHASE
- Lymphadenopathy
- Anemia
- Depression
- Anorexia
- Fever
- Weight loss
- Ocular and nasal discharge
- Dyspnea
- Edema (extremities and scrotum)

SUBCLINICAL PHASE
- Few clinical signs
- CNS symptoms

CHRONIC PHASE
- Severe weight loss
- Debilitation
- Anterior uveitis
- Retinal hemorrhage
- CNS signs
- Secondary bacterial infections
- Bleeding tendencies

DIAGNOSIS
- Positive indirect immunofluorescent antibody test
- Complete blood count:
    Pancytopenia (25% of patients)
    Nonregenerative anemia
    Thrombocytopenia
- Serum chemistry: Hyperglobulinemia

TREATMENT

- Tetracycline: 22 mg/kg t.i.d. for 14 days
- Doxycycline: 10 mg/kg q 14 days
- Supportive care will be required for some animals:
    IV fluid therapy
    Blood transfusions
    Anabolic steroids
- For recurrent infections, tetracycline 6.6 mg/kg daily for long term

 TECH ALERT

Infection with *E. canis* produces no long-term immunity.

CANINE GRANULOCYTIC EHRLICHIOSIS (GE)

Two forms of this disease exist: canine granulocytic ehrlichiosis (GE) caused by *E. ewingii* and canine GE caused by *E. equi*. Dogs infected by *E. ewingii* present with acute polyarthritis and inflammatory joint disease. This syndrome is linked to the tick *Amblyomma americanum* as its vector, and it is not seasonal. Dogs infected with *E. equi* present with nonspecific signs of severe lethargy and anorexia. This disease is seasonal and corresponds to the peak feeding season of the vector *Ixodes dammini,* the deer tick.

CLINICAL SIGNS

E. EWINGII

- Sudden onset of fever
- Lethargy
- Anorexia
- Lameness
- Muscular stiffness

E. EQUI

- Acute onset of fever
- Severe, often debilitating lethargy
- Anorexia

DIAGNOSIS

E. EWINGII

- Complete blood count:
    Mild, nonregenerative anemia

Thrombocytopenia
Monocytosis
Eosinophilia
Morulae in neutrophils (1% to 9%)
- Serum chemistries: Increased ALT
- Positive *E. canis* test

E. EQUI
- Complete blood count:
  Thrombocytopenia
  Lymphopenia
- Serum chemistries:
  Increased ALP (100%)
  Increased amylase (50%)
  Hypoalbuminemia
- Urine: Proteinuria
- Positive *E. canis* test

TREATMENT
- Tetracycline: 22 mg/kg t.i.d. q 14 days
- Doxycycline: 10 mg/kg q 12 h for 7 to 10 days
- Supportive care if required

INFORMATION FOR CLIENTS
- Ticks present a disease threat for pets and humans.
- The prognosis for these syndromes is good.
- Clinical signs should improve within 48 hours from the start of treatment.
- Check pets frequently for ticks, and remove the ticks when found.
- Avoid tick-infested areas. Do not expose yourself to the blood from the tick.

LYME DISEASE (BORRELIOSIS)

Lyme borreliosis is a complex, multiorgan disorder caused by the spirochete *Borrelia burgdorferi*. The spirochete is passed to the host animal or human through the bite of a tick in the genus *Ixodes*. Ticks must remain attached to the host for a minimum of 48 hours for infection to occur. Although the disease is worldwide in distribution, it is endemic in most of the northeastern states, with approximately 90% of all cases occurring in New York, New Jersey, Connecticut, and Pennsylvania. (Zoonosis—same ticks transmit to humans in contaminated environment.)

Symptoms include dermatologic, arthritic, cardiac, and neurologic abnormalities. Some animals may develop a severe nephritis (especially Labrador Retrievers). Signs may appear months after the tick bite and may be vague and nonspecific, making diagnosis difficult. Animals spending time outdoors in tick-infested areas are at the greatest risk of infection.

Diagnosis is based on clinical signs and a positive ELISA or antibody titer. (It may be difficult to evaluate titers when dogs have been vaccinated.) Doxycycline is the drug of choice for the treatment of borreliosis. Antibiotic therapy may *not* eliminate the organism from the infected animal, and some animals may be permanently infected leading to chronic cases with flare-ups.

CLINICAL SIGNS
- Fever
- Anorexia
- Lethargy
- Lymphadenopathy
- Episodic lameness
- Presence or absence of myocardial abnormalities
- Rash around the tick bite
- Nephritis (especially in Labrador Retrievers)

DIAGNOSIS
- No specific hematological or biochemical changes have been noted except where specific organ systems are involved.
- Synovial fluid: Suppurative polyarthritis (increased numbers of nucleated cells)
- Antibody titers >64 may indicate infection
- Positive ELISA test

TREATMENT
- Doxycycline: 10 mg/kg PO q 24 h for 21 to 28 days
- Antiinflammatory drugs for pain:
    Aspirin: 25 to 35 mg/kg PO q 8 h
    Prednisolone: 0.25 mg/kg/day

- Vaccination of seronegative dogs is recommended in endemic areas (LymeVax, Ft. Dodge). Vaccination of seropositive dogs or dogs not in endemic areas is not recommended.

⊕ TECH ALERT
No antibiotic is 100% effective in eliminating the organism.

INFORMATION FOR CLIENTS
- Animal infection should alert owners to the possibility of human infection from ticks in the environment.
- Infected animals may have relapses of symptoms even after treatment.
- Vaccination of dogs already exposed to *B. burgdorferi* is ineffective.
- Avoid exposure to environments where high concentrations of ticks might be found.
- Use a tick collar or other means of tick repellent for animals traveling to infested areas.

THE REPRODUCTIVE SYSTEM

The female reproductive system consists of two ovaries and the female duct system, including the oviducts, uterus, cervix, vagina, and vulva (Fig. 11-1). The primary functions of this system are to provide eggs for fertilization and to protect the developing embryo during pregnancy. All of these structures are composed of tissue that is sensitive to hormones produced by the female.

Hormones such as estrogen and progesterone act on the reproductive system to prepare it for pregnancy and to maintain that pregnancy. When the response to these hormones is abnormal, disease can result. Although not technically a part of the female reproductive system, the mammary glands are also reactive to hormonal abnormalities, and diseases involving them are frequently seen in small animal practice.

The male reproductive system consists of two testicles and the male duct system, including the urethra, prostate gland, and penis (Fig. 11-2). Other structures often involved with disease processes are the scrotum and the prepuce. The main hormonal influence in the male is testosterone, although abnormal estrogen levels can also affect the male reproductive system.

Diseases involving the reproductive system are frequently seen in veterinary practice. These include vaginal disorders, uterine disorders, pregnancy disorders, lactation disorders, disease of the prostate, and neoplasia of the genital system and mammary glands.

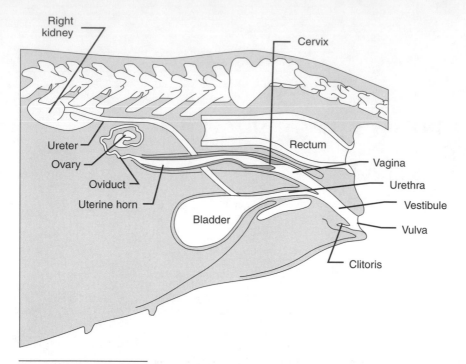

FIGURE 11-1. Female urinary and reproductive organs of bitch (lateral view). (From Colville T, Bassert JM: *Clinical anatomy and physiology for veterinary technicians,* St Louis, 2002, Mosby.)

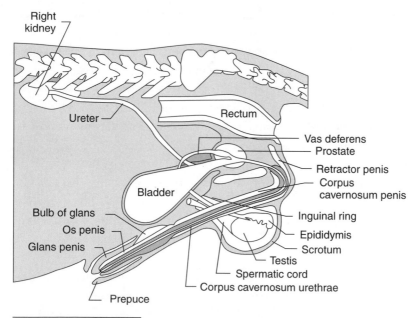

FIGURE 11-2. Male urinary and reproductive organs of dog (lateral view). (From Colville T, Bassert JM: *Clinical anatomy and physiology for veterinary technicians,* St Louis, 2002, Mosby.)

FEMALE REPRODUCTIVE DISEASE

VAGINAL DISORDERS

VAGINITIS

Vaginitis is a fairly common occurrence in prepuberal bitches. The most common sign of juvenile (puppy) vaginitis is vulvar discharge. This condition responds well to systemic antibiotic therapy and usually resolves after the first estrous cycle. Adult vaginitis can be the result of a variety of factors. Anatomic abnormalities, bacterial infection, traumatic injuries, or chemical irritation can all result in vaginal inflammation. Viral vaginitis also occurs in conjunction with canine herpesvirus infections.

PYOMETRA

Pyometra is also frequently seen in small animal medicine. Increasing levels of progesterone following ovulation results in hyperplasia and hypertrophy of the endometrial glands of the uterus. Inappropriate response results in cystic endometrial hyperplasia with accumulation of fluid within the uterine lumen. Progesterone also produces a decrease in myometrial contractions and predisposes the uterus to secondary bacterial infection (pyometra). The most common microorganism isolated in pyometra is *Escherichia coli,* although *Staphylococcus* spp., *Streptococcus* spp., *Klebsiella, Pasteurella, Proteus,* and *Moraxella* have also been implicated.

The development of pyometra seems to be the final stage of a continuum beginning with endometrial hyperplasia and progressing through cystic endometrial hyperplasia and endometritis. Animals presented for treatment tend to be middle age or older, within 60 days of their last estrous cycle.

CLINICAL SIGNS
- Vulvar discharge
- Abdominal enlargement
- Vomiting
- Lethargy
- Polyuria/polydipsia
- Dehydration
- Azotemia

DIAGNOSIS

- Radiology indicates an enlarged uterus (must rule out pregnancy).
- Ultrasound examination can distinguish between fluid and pregnancy.
- Complete blood count (CBC) shows leukocytosis, neutrophilia with a left shift, and dehydration. A nonregenerative anemia may be seen.
- Serum chemistry may show:
    Increased alkaline phosphatase levels
    Increased serum protein
    Increased blood urea nitrogen
- Vaginal cytology shows degenerative neutrophils, endometrial cells, and bacteria.
- Culture and sensitivity should be performed if medical treatment is to be attempted or if the animal is systemically ill.

TREATMENT

- Ovariohysterectomy is the preferred treatment for pyometra.
- Dehydration and azotemia must be corrected before surgery.
- If the animal is used for breeding, owners may elect medical treatment:
    Prostaglandin $F_2\alpha$ (Lutylase): 0.1 to 0.25 mg/kg SQ 1 to 2 times daily for 3 to 5 days or until the uterus is empty. Side effects seen with prostaglandin infection usually resolve within 60 minutes of injection (e.g., sweating, panting, salivation, vomiting/defecation, urination).
    Systemic broad-spectrum antibiotics should be given until culture results come back from the laboratory.

INFORMATION FOR CLIENTS

- Ovariohysterectomy (spaying) prevents this disease.
- Early and aggressive treatment is important.
- The treatment of choice for pyometra is ovariohysterectomy (even in older dogs and cats).
- Approximately 26% to 40% of bitches have a recurrence of pyometra within 1 year of medical treatment.
- Medical treatment is more successful when the cervix is open and draining.
- In bitches with pyometra, 5% to 8% mortality is associated with ovariohysterectomy.

PREGNANCY DISORDERS

Disorders of pregnancy include fetal death and abortion/reabsorption, dystocia, inappropriate maternal behavior, mastitis, and puerperal tetany. Although there are other problems associated with pregnancy and parturition, these are the most commonly seen problems in small animal medicine. The normal gestation period for the dog and cat is between 62 and 65 days. Fetuses can be palpated about 25 to 36 days after breeding in the dog, and 21 to 28 days in the cat. Fetal skeletal mineralization can be detected radiographically at 45 days of gestation. Ultrasonography can provide information on the status of the fetuses after about 20 days. It is difficult to determine the number of fetuses, especially in large litters.

Fetal deaths early in gestation result in reabsorption with no expulsion of uterine contents. Owners may report that the animal has "failed to conceive" after what they consider a successful breeding. Organisms such as *Brucella canis,* canine herpesvirus, FIP, FeLV, and panleukopenia can produce fetal death or abortion.

Dystocia can be defined as difficulty in delivery of fetuses through the birth canal. The causes of dystocia can be divided into fetal factors, maternal factors, and combinations of both. Fetal factors include large fetuses (large puppy or kitten, fetal anasarca, or hydrocephalus) and abnormal positioning (transverse presentation). Breech presentation is *not* an abnormality in the bitch or queen. Maternal factors include a narrowed birth canal (developmental or trauma related) and uterine inertia (lack of coordinated contractions or exhaustion of the uterine musculature from prolonged contractions).

DYSTOCIA

CLINICAL SIGNS
- A bitch or queen has been in labor longer than 4 hours without producing a fetus.
- A green vaginal discharge develops during parturition.
- More than one hour has elapsed between births.

DIAGNOSIS
- Physical examination with digital palpation of vagina
- Radiography to evaluate the fetal position, size, and number
- Ultrasonography to evaluate fetal viability and distress

TREATMENT

- Manual manipulation: a fetus lodged in the vaginal canal can be manually dislodged through careful manipulation.
- Oxytocin 1.1 to 2.2 IU/kg can be used to correct secondary inertia.
- If medical treatment fails to correct the situation, a cesarean section is recommended.

INFORMATION FOR CLIENTS

- Owners should prepare a whelping box for the animal, and make sure the animal is comfortable sleeping in that box before whelping.
- Nutrition of the pregnant animal is important, with increased demands being placed on the mother as the litter develops.
- During the birthing process, owners should be advised to closely supervise the animal but not hover around, creating stress for the mother. Children and other pets should be kept out of the area.
- If labor and delivery are not progressing steadily, veterinary help should be obtained.
- Owners can predict parturition by monitoring the rectal temperature of the animal. Rectal temperature usually drops below 100 F° 24 hours before the beginning of labor.
- After a cesarean section, owners may have to support the neonates until the mother is fully recovered.
- Ovariohysterectomy can be performed at the same time as the cesarean section in animals not used for breeding.

INAPPROPRIATE MATERNAL BEHAVIOR

Appropriate maternal behavior is important to the survival and development of neonates. Nursing, retrieving, grooming, and protecting are all considered normal behavior. The dam should demonstrate caution when moving about the whelping box; she should lie quietly while the neonates nurse. Because puppies and kittens do not have the ability to thermoregulate their body temperature in the first few weeks of life, the mother is responsible for keeping them warm. Grooming is important to stimulate cardiovascular and respiratory function, to stimulate elimination, and to remove waste material from the coat. Some dams, however, display increased protective behavior or fear-induced behaviors. Some cannibalize their litters. When these inappropriate behaviors occur, it is up to the owner to intervene and protect the health and well-being of the neonates.

CLINICAL SIGNS

- Mother is restless (will not stay in the box with the puppies or kittens).
- Neonates are constantly crying.
- Mother is actively attacking and killing her young. Owners may not directly see such acts; however, the number of neonates will be seen to decrease.

DIAGNOSIS

- Observation of mother

TREATMENT

- Tranquilization of the mother:
    Acepromazine: 0.01 to 0.02 mg/kg
    Diazepam: 0.5 to 2.4 mg/kg PO (canine); 1 to 2 mg/cat (feline)

INFORMATION FOR CLIENTS

- Do not use affected bitches for breeding.
- Do not leave puppies unattended with an affected bitch.

LACTATION DISORDERS

The mammary gland achieves its maximum growth and development during pregnancy. The decline in progesterone levels before parturition results in the synthesis of enzymes that permit lactogenesis. Oxytocin released in response to suckling increases milk letdown within the gland. *Agalactia,* lack of milk production, can result from stress, malnutrition, premature parturition, or infection.

Galactostasis, or milk stasis, can result in painful engorgement of the mammary glands, and *mastitis,* a septic inflammation of the mammary gland, occurs in pet animals. Mastitis is probably seen more commonly in the bitch and queen than the other two problems. Mastitis may be acute or chronic and may involve one or more of the mammary glands.

CLINICAL SIGNS

- Mammary discomfort
- Discolored milk
- Fever
- Reluctance to allow nursing
- Abscessed glands

TREATMENT
- Broad-spectrum systemic antibiotic:
    Cephalexin: 5.5 to 16.5 mg/kg PO q 8 h
    Clavamox: 15.4 mg/kg PO q 8 to 12 h
- Administer warm compresses, then milk the affected glands.
- Protect the affected gland(s) from trauma.

INFORMATION FOR CLIENTS
- Mastitis can recur in subsequent lactations.
- Prophylactic use of antibiotics is not advocated.
- Puppies and kittens should not be allowed to nurse from affected glands but can continue to use the noninfected teats.

PROSTATIC DISEASES

Although both dogs and cats have prostate glands, prostatic disease is much more common in the canine. The canine prostate gland is the only accessory sex gland in the dog. The gland is located just caudal to the bladder, encircling the proximal urethra at the neck of the bladder. The size and position of the gland changes with the age of the dog so that the gland is mostly abdominal over the age of 5 years. The purpose of the prostate gland is to produce fluid as a transport and support medium for sperm during ejaculation.

The prostate increases in size and weight as the dog matures. Dogs castrated before maturity have normal prostatic growth totally inhibited. When adult dogs are castrated, the prostate undergoes involution.

Clinical diseases associated with the prostate include benign hyperplasia, cysts, prostatitis, abscessation, and neoplasia. Clinical signs of prostatic disease are similar regardless of the cause. Accurate diagnosis depends on a good physical examination, laboratory evaluation, and biopsy.

BENIGN PROSTATIC HYPERPLASIA

Benign prostatic hyperplasia is an aging change that occurs in dogs as early as 2.5 years of age. The condition is associated with an altered androgen/estrogen ratio and requires the presence of the testes. Although the size increases with hyperplasia, secretory function decreases. Blood supply to the gland increases, and the gland tends to bleed easily. Most dogs have no clinical signs.

CLINICAL SIGNS
- May be asymptomatic
- Tenesmus
- Prostate palpates symmetrically (enlarged and nonpainful)

DIAGNOSIS
- A physical examination is recommended.
- Biopsy provides the only accurate diagnosis.

TREATMENT
- Castration results in a 70% decrease in size of the gland within 7 to 14 days.
- Low-dose estrogen therapy: Diethylstilbestrol 0.2 to 1 mg/day for 5 days. Potential side effects must be considered when selecting estrogen therapy (bone marrow suppression).
- Flutamide: 5 mg/kg/day (not approved for veterinary use and is expensive).
- Megestrol acetate: 0.55 mg/kg/day for 4 weeks (this drug is not approved for use in male dogs).

INFORMATION FOR CLIENTS
- Early castration prevents this condition.
- Castration, even in the older animal, alleviates this condition.
- Drug therapy results in temporary improvement, but the condition will recur when drug therapy is discontinued.

PROSTATITIS

The prostate gland is predisposed to bacterial infection through the urinary system as well as direct infection of the gland itself. *Escherichia coli* is the most frequently isolated bacterial organism involved in canine prostatitis. Other gram-negative microorganisms, such as *Proteus, Klebsiella, Pseudomonas, Streptococcus, Staphylococcus,* and *Brucella canis,* have also been found to cause this disease. Bacterial prostatitis may be acute or chronic and affects sexually mature male dogs.

CLINICAL SIGNS

ACUTE PROSTATITIS

- Anorexia
- Fever
- Lethargy
- Stiff gait in the rear limbs
- Caudal abdominal pain

CHRONIC PROSTATITIS

- May be asymptomatic
- History of chronic, periodic urinary tract infections

DIAGNOSIS

- Urinalysis: Urine shows blood, increased white blood cell (WBC) count, and the presence of bacteria.
- Physical examination
- Urine culture

TREATMENT

- Antibiotic therapy should be instituted for 28 days (acute form). (For the chronic form use same antibiotic therapy regimen for at least 6 weeks.) The choice of antibiotic should be based on culture and sensitivity results and may be started IV if the animal is in serious condition:
  - Enrofloxacin: 5 mg/kg q 12 h
  - Trimethoprim/sulfonamide: 15.4 mg/kg q12 h
  - Erythromycin: 9.9 mg/kg q 8 h
  - Chloramphenicol: 30 to 55 mg/kg q 8 h
  - Ciprofloxacin: 4.4 to 8.8 mg/kg q 12 h
- Castration
- Prostatectomy, a difficult surgery with serious postsurgical side effects, can be considered.

INFORMATION FOR CLIENTS

- Long-term antibiotic therapy is essential to control this disease.
- Prolonged use of antibiotics requires monitoring with prostatic fluid cultures and examinations to ensure that toxic side effects do not develop.
- Castration may be beneficial.

PROSTATIC ABSCESSATION

Prostatic abscessation is a serious form of bacterial prostatitis in which pockets of purulent exudate develop within the gland. The disease may present with systemic signs.

CLINICAL SIGNS
- Tenesmus
- Urethral discharge
- Lethargy
- Pain
- Vomiting
- Hematuria
- Fever
- Depression

DIAGNOSIS
- History and physical examination
- CBC and serum chemistries
- Leukocytosis or normal WBC
- Liver enzymes may be elevated
- Hypoglycemia
- Hypokalemia
- Prostatic aspiration—hemorrhagic, purulent, septic

TREATMENT
- Surgical drainage is the treatment of choice.
- Castration
- Antibiotic therapy
- IV fluid therapy (in cases of sepsis or peritonitis)

INFORMATION FOR CLIENTS
- These cases are expensive and difficult to treat.
- Survival is approximately 50% after 1 year.

PROSTATIC NEOPLASIA

This condition is uncommon in the dog but has been seen in the cat. Prostatic neoplasia can develop in both intact and neutered male dogs. All neoplasms that affect the prostate are malignant. Clinical signs are similar to other prostatic diseases. Treatment is unrewarding, and a cure is unlikely.

NEOPLASIA OF THE GENITAL SYSTEM AND THE MAMMARY GLANDS

Tumors of the male genital tract include those of the testicles, prostate, penis, prepuce, and scrotum.

TESTICULAR TUMORS

Approximately 5% to 15% of all tumors seen in the male dog are testicular tumors. Cryptorchid dogs and dogs with inguinal hernias are at greatest risk of testicular tumors; tumor development is twice as common in testicles retained in the inguinal canal as those within the abdomen. These tumors are usually seen in older, intact male dogs (9 to 12 years). Testicular tumors in the cat are uncommon.

CLINICAL SIGNS
- Older, intact male dogs (9 to 12 years) are predisposed to this condition.
- Nonpainful testicular enlargement may be seen.
- Feminization (bilateral nonpruritic alopecia, hyperpigmentation in the inguinal region, gynecomastia, nonregenerative anemia, and thrombocytopenia) occurs in approximately 25% to 50% of dogs with Sertoli cell tumors.
- Enlarged lymph nodes may be seen in some animals (10% to 20%).

DIAGNOSIS
- Clinical signs

TREATMENT
- Castration is the treatment of choice.
- If adjunct treatment is required, chemotherapy and radiation therapy can be used.
- Whole blood transfusion should be performed if the animal is myelosuppressed.

INFORMATION FOR CLIENTS
- Castration of male dogs at an early age prevents this disease.
- Dogs with myelosuppression from excess estrogen levels may need a whole blood transfusion.

PENILE, PREPUCIAL, AND SCROTAL TUMORS

Penile tumors in the dog and cat are rare. The most commonly seen neoplasia involving the penis and the prepuce is the transmissible veneral tumor (TVT). This tumor occurs only in the canine. It is most commonly seen in temperate climates and in areas having large free-roaming dog populations. It is spread during sexual contact and can be transmitted by licking and sniffing.

CLINICAL SIGNS
- These tumors are found on sexually intact male and female dogs.
- Cauliflower-like masses appear at the base of the penis or on the lining of the prepuce; they are seen on the vulva in the female (tumors are friable and bleed easily).
- Lesions may also be seen on the face and rectum.

DIAGNOSIS
- Cytology: Imprint smears reveal large, round-to-oval cells with abundant pale cytoplasm containing many vacuoles; the nuclei contain frequent mitotic figures and visible nucleoli.

TREATMENT
- TVTs are immunogenic and may spontaneously regress with adequate tumor stimulation.
- Chemotherapy: Vincristine therapy (0.025 mg/kg IV once weekly) cures over 90% of cases. Treatment should continue for 2 weeks after resolution of the tumor (generally 4 to 6 treatments).
- Surgical removal of small, localized lesions is recommended.

TUMORS OF THE FEMALE GENITAL TRACT

Tumors of the female genital tract include ovarian tumors, uterine and cervical tumors, vaginal and vulval neoplasia, and tumors of the mammary glands.

Tumors of the ovaries and uterus are uncommon in both dogs and cats. Surgical removal of these tumors is the treatment of choice. Vaginal and vulvar tumors are the most common tumors of the female genital tract in the canine. They are uncommon in the cat.

CLINICAL SIGNS
- A pedunculated mass protruding from the vulva may be seen.
- Perineal swelling, vaginal discharge, dysuria, or constipation may be seen.

DIAGNOSIS
- Clinical signs

TREATMENT
- Surgical removal with ovariohysterectomy reduces recurrence.

INFORMATION FOR CLIENTS
- Most of these tumors are benign.
- The prognosis is good for this tumor.

MAMMARY TUMORS

Tumors of the mammary gland are the most common tumor of female dogs, representing approximately 50% of all tumors of female dogs. They are the third most common tumor of female cats. These are usually tumors of older animals. The tumors are hormone-dependent in the canine but less so in the feline. The risk of mammary tumor is 0.5% for bitches spayed before their first estrus, 8% for those spayed after one estrous cycle, and 26% for bitches spayed after two or more cycles. Risk in the cat is similar for spayed and nonspayed females.

Approximately 50% of canine mammary tumors are benign. In the cat, only 10% to 20% are benign. Tumors may be singular or multiple, occurring in any of the glands.

Malignant and benign tumors may occur simultaneously. Both tumor types can occur as firm, well-demarcated lesions, so it is impossible to distinguish malignant from benign lesions by appearance. Rapid growth, local tissue invasion, and ulceration are usually hallmarks of malignant tumors. In the dog and the cat, tumor size is probably the best prognostic indicator, whereas factors such as age of the patient, tumor numbers, and tumor location have less prognostic value.

CLINICAL SIGNS
- Firm nodule is palpable in the mammary chain or gland.
- Surrounding tissue may be involved; lymph nodes in the region may be enlarged.

DIAGNOSIS
- Physical examination
- CBC, serum chemistries, and thoracic radiographs should be evaluated before surgery.

TREATMENT
- Any accepted method of surgical removal may be used. The surgeon should choose the simplest procedure that removes the entire tumor.
- Chemotherapy may have minimal antitumor activity in both the canine and the feline.
- Adjunct chemotherapy may be used along with surgery. Doxorubicin or dactinomycin may be used in the dog; doxorubicin and cyclophosphamide may be used in cats (doxorubicin 30 mg/m^2 IV q 21 days; dactinomycin 0.7 mg/m^2 q 21 days; cyclophosphamide 100 mg/m^2 PO once daily on days 3, 4, 5, 6 after doxorubicin).

INFORMATION FOR CLIENTS
- Veterinarians cannot distinguish benign tumors from malignant ones without biopsies. Surgical removal is advised for all mammary tumors, followed by histology.
- In cats with tumors less than 2 cm, survival times of up to 3 years have been reported; larger masses usually mean shorter survival times.
- Eighty percent to ninety percent of all feline mammary tumors are malignant, whereas only 50% of canine tumors are malignant.
- In animals, chemotherapy is not curative for this type of tumor.
- Although ovariohysterectomy has not been proven to increase survival, it is recommended because 50% to 60% of canine mammary tumors have estrogen receptors on their cells that may increase the recurrence of tumors.

twelve

DISEASES OF THE
RESPIRATORY SYSTEM

All of the cells within an animal's body require oxygen for metabolism. When glucose is burned (in the cell) with oxygen, the by-products are energy, water, and carbon dioxide. Carbon dioxide, a waste product, must be eliminated from the body, whereas water and energy are used to maintain all the life processes. The respiratory system transports oxygen to the bloodstream and removes carbon dioxide. Malfunction of this system affects all functions in the living animal.

We can arbitrarily divide the respiratory system into the *upper respiratory tract* (nasal cavity, sinuses, nasopharynx, and larynx) (Fig. 12-1) and the *lower respiratory tract* (trachea, bronchi, lungs, and pleural cavity) (Fig. 12-2). The technology student is referred to an anatomy text for review of the anatomy and physiology of the respiratory system.

DISEASES OF THE UPPER RESPIRATORY TRACT

Diseases of the upper respiratory system include rhinitis, nasal tumors, epistaxis, sinusitis, tonsillitis, and laryngitis.

Although upper airway disease is not nearly as common in dogs and cats as it is in humans, it is still seen clinically and causes concern for owners.

RHINITIS

CLINICAL SIGNS
- Serous, mucoid, or mucopurulent nasal discharge
- Sneezing, pawing at nose

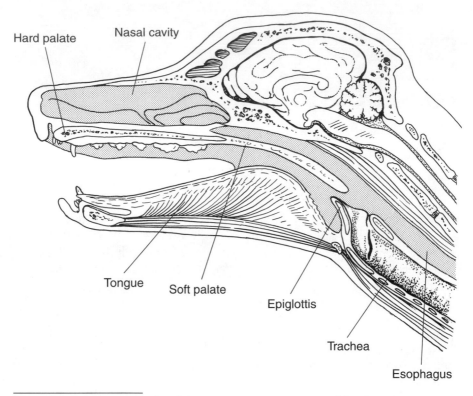

FIGURE 12-1.   Cross-section of the upper respiratory tract of the dog. (From McBride DF: *Learning veterinary terminology,* ed 2, St Louis, 2002, Mosby.)

- Coughing or gagging
- Encrustation on nares
- Rarely presents as single disease (usually appears as sequela to other respiratory infections)

DIAGNOSIS
- Clinical signs
- Culture and sensitivity results show *Staphylococcus* strains

TREATMENT
- Clean the nares gently, and apply a soothing ointment.
- Administer systemic antibiotics if necessary.

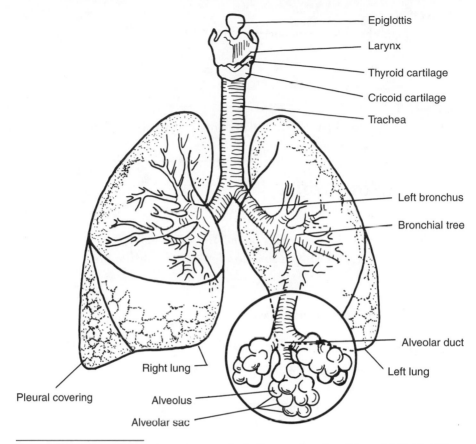

FIGURE 12-2.   Lower respiratory tract, including an alveolus. (From McBride DF: *Learning veterinary terminology,* ed 2, St Louis, 2002, Mosby.)

- Administer vasoconstrictive drugs in combination with antihistamines to clear the nasal cavity.
    Neosynephrine drops: place several drops in each nostril 3 to 4 times daily.
    Ephedrine: 1 to 2 mg/kg PO q 8 to 12 h

NASAL TUMORS

CLINICAL SIGNS

- Unilateral mucoid nasal discharge unresponsive to therapy
- Nasal hemorrhage
- Sneezing (uncommon)

DIAGNOSIS
- Radiographs to locate the mass
- Endoscopy
- Biopsy

TREATMENT
- Surgical removal (surgery is usually only palliative)
- Masses usually recur

EPISTAXIS (NOSEBLEED)

CLINICAL SIGNS
- Bleeding from the nares (may be unilateral or bilateral)
- Usually associated with trauma, foreign objects, or tumors

DIAGNOSIS
- Fresh blood from the nasal cavity

TREATMENT
- Locate the exact site of bleeding in the nasal cavity
- Stop the bleeding:
    Vasoconstrictive drugs instilled into the nasal cavity
    Apply pressure to the area if possible
    Vitamin K therapy (if coagulation is a problem)

SINUSITIS

This condition usually involves the frontal or maxillary sinus in the dog and manifests as a collection of pus in the area, resulting in a swelling over the sinus. The most common cause of this problem in the dog is tooth root abscess.

CLINICAL SIGNS
- Swelling under the eye on the side of the bad tooth
- Unilateral nasal discharge

DIAGNOSIS
- Examination of the nasal and oral cavity
- Radiographs to determine whether there is resorption of bone
- Culture and sensitivity of all fistula tracts

TREATMENT
- Antibiotics (based on culture and sensitivity results)
- Removal of the infected tooth to promote drainage
- Flushing of fistula tracts with antiseptic solution

TONSILLITIS

Tonsils are the "sentinels" of the respiratory tract, providing lymphoid protection to the lower respiratory system pathway. When invaded by infectious agents the tonsils hypertrophy, resulting in difficulty swallowing and sore throats. Neoplasia involving the tonsils is fairly common in domestic animals.

CLINICAL SIGNS
- Anorexia
- Increased salivation
- Pain on opening the mouth

DIAGNOSIS
- Visual examination shows inflamed, swollen tonsils.
- Tonsils may be coated with mucus or pus or have abscesses on the surface.

TREATMENT
- Systemic antibiotics
- Soft or liquid diet
- Medication for pain relief: NSAIDs such as aspirin 10 to 25 mg/kg PO q 8 to 12 h (dogs); 10 mg/kg q.o.d. (cats)
- Surgical removal in cases of chronic infection or neoplasia

LARYNGITIS

Although the most common cause of laryngitis is excessive barking, howling, or meowing, infection from high in the respiratory tract can spread to the larynx, resulting in the loss of voice.

CLINICAL SIGNS
- Loss of voice or alteration in quality of voice
- Cough
- Increased concentration of mucus in the back of the throat

TECH ALERT

Handle all animals with a history of voice change with care. Rabies can also cause a change in vocal quality.

DIAGNOSIS
- History
- Physical examination: Red, inflamed throat

TREATMENT
- Restrict barking or meowing
- Antibiotics (if infection is part of symptoms)
- Antiinflammatory medication: Glucocorticoids 0.5 to 1 mg/kg per day; taper dose after 7 days

INFORMATION FOR CLIENTS
- Upper airway diseases are usually self-limiting.
- Tumors of the nasal cavity and tonsils are most commonly squamous cell carcinomas.
- In most cases, treatment is aimed at making the animal more comfortable. In cases of infection, antibiotics may be required for several weeks.

DISEASES OF THE LOWER RESPIRATORY TRACT

Diseases involving the lower respiratory tract are of more serious clinical significance than those of the upper airways. Examples of lower airway diseases include tracheobronchitis, tracheal collapse, feline asthma, feline viral respiratory infections, pneumonia, heartworm disease (feline), neoplasia, pulmonary edema, and hemothorax/pneumothorax.

INFECTIOUS CANINE TRACHEOBRONCHITIS (KENNEL COUGH)

This disease syndrome involves a collection of agents including viruses, bacteria, mycoplasmas, fungi, and parasites. Some of the most commonly incriminated agents are canine parainfluenza virus, canine adenovirus, canine herpesvirus, reovirus, *Bordetella bronchiseptica*, mycoplasma, and occasionally the canine distemper virus.

CLINICAL SIGNS
- A history of exposure to other animals at a kennel, hospital, grooming facility, or show
- A dry, hacking, paroxysmal cough (except for cough, a normal, healthy-looking animal)

DIAGNOSIS
- Clinical signs and history
- Cough on tracheal palpation in an otherwise healthy dog

TREATMENT
- Administer antibiotics if any deeper respiratory involvement is found or if animal is febrile (base choice on culture and sensitivity results).
    - Novobiocin/tetracycline/prednisolone combination (Delta-Alba-plex, Upjohn): 22 mg/kg PO q 12 h
- Glucocorticoids:
    - Temeril-P: 1 tablet/9 kg q 12 h
    - Prednisone, prednisolone: 0.25 to 0.5 mg/kg b.i.d. for 5 to 7 days, then taper dose
- Antitussives:
    - Hycodan (5 mg hydrocodone bitartrate): 0.22 mg/kg PO b.i.d. to q.i.d.
    - Codeine: 1.1 to 2.2 mg/kg q 6 to 8 h
    - Torbutrol: 0.55 mg/kg q 6 to 12 h
- Bronchial dilators:
    - Aminophylline: 11 mg/kg PO q 6 to 12 h
    - Terbutaline (Brethine): 1.25 to 5 mg PO q 8 to 12 h

INFORMATION FOR CLIENTS
- This is a self-limiting disease. It can take 2 to 3 weeks to resolve.
- Treatment is aimed at making the animal (and often the owner) more comfortable.
- Vaccination with an injectable vaccine should be obtained 2 to 3 weeks before boarding or possible exposure to the disease. Intranasal vaccine can be given closer to the time of exposure. Vaccination significantly reduces the severity of the disease.

Collapsing Trachea

The etiology of this disease is not entirely known; however, a reduction in the glycoprotein and glycosaminoglycan content of the hyaline cartilage of the tracheal rings is a constant finding in dogs affected by this syndrome. This syndrome is frequently seen in middle age to old, obese toy and miniature breeds but can also be seen in young animals (Yorkies seem to be overrepresented). The defect involves tracheal rings that lose their ability to remain firm, subsequently collapsing during respiration.

CLINICAL SIGNS
- History of paroxysmal cough (harsh, dry, "goose honk" cough)
- Cough often worse on exercise or excitement or when pulling on the collar
- Often concurrent signs of heart disease

DIAGNOSIS
- Tracheal palpation elicits a "goose honk" cough.
- All other physical examination parameters may be normal.
- Radiography on static views may or may not show an alteration in the contour of the trachea. Dorsoventral (DV) and lateral views (both inspiratory and expiratory) are necessary to see this condition.
- Endoscopy demonstrates the actual ring collapsing when the animal breathes.
- Ultrasound provides real-time pictures of collapse.
- Fluoroscopy shows collapse on respirations.
- Rule out all other causes of cough.

TREATMENT
Symptomatic treatment
- Treatment to slow breathing in acute cases:
    Acepromazine: 0.02 to 0.2 mg/kg IV, IM, SC
    Oxygen therapy (mask) or intubation
    Dexamethasone: 1 mg/kg IV
    Butorphanol: 0.05 to 0.1 mg/kg IV, IM, SC, q 6 to 12 h
- Treatment to slow breathing in chronic cases:
    Antitussives:
    Hycodan (5 mg hydrocodone bitartrate): 0.22 mg/kg PO b.i.d. to q.i.d.

Butorphanol: 0.5 to 0.1 mg/kg PO q 12 h

Lomotil: 0.2 to 0.5 mg PO q 12 h (unproven drug for this purpose in the United States; this product contains atropine, which can cause constipation)

Glucocorticoids:

Prednisolone: 0.5 mg/kg PO q 12 h; taper dose after 7 to 10 days

*Bronchial dilators:**

Theophylline: 20 mg/kg PO q 12 h

Terbutaline (Brethine, Ciba): 1.25 to 5 mg/dog PO q 8 to 12 h

SURGICAL TREATMENT

- Keep the trachea open with the insertion of external prosthetic supports.
- Surgical correction involves a number of possible complications, making the procedure unrewarding.

INFORMATION FOR CLIENTS

- Once this condition develops, it requires life-long management.
- Treatment is aimed at reducing inflammation in the airway and making the animal more comfortable.
- Management techniques that help include the following:
    Aggressive weight reduction
    Decreased exposure to inhaled irritants such as cigarette smoke
    Use of a harness instead of a collar for restraint
    Aggressive treatment of respiratory infections
    Monitoring and treatment of congestive heart failure if it develops

FELINE ASTHMA

Feline asthma, as in human asthma, is a disease characterized by spontaneous bronchoconstriction, airway inflammation, and airway hyperreactivity. Clinical signs of feline asthma include coughing, wheezing, and labored breathing, usually of acute onset.

In affected cats airway epithelium may hypertrophy, goblet cells and submucosal glands may produce excessive amounts of mucus, and the bronchial mucosa may become infiltrated with inflammatory cells. All of these

---

*Bronchial dilators act to decrease intrathoracic pressures during expiration, thereby decreasing the collapse of the tracheal membrane.

changes result in decreased airflow. A 50% decrease in the lumen of the airway results in a 16-fold decrease in the amount of air moving through the system.

It would seem that chronic airway inflammation plays an important role in feline asthma. Decreasing inflammation in the airways and improving airflow are the primary goals of treatment.

CLINICAL SIGNS

- Acute onset of labored breathing
- Cough (may be chronic)
- Wheeze
- Lethargy

DIAGNOSIS

- No physical examination findings are diagnostic for feline asthma.
- Clinical signs and history help establish diagnosis.
- Radiographs may show signs of diffuse prominent bronchial markings consistent with airway inflammation (often described as "doughnuts").

TREATMENT

- Manage airway inflammation with high-dose, long-term corticosteroid therapy:
    - Prednisone: 1 to 2 mg/kg PO q 12 h for 10 to 14 days, then slowly taper over 2 to 3 months
    - DepoMedrol: 10 to 20 mg IM q 2 to 4 weeks (if unable to dose orally)
- Bronchodilators:
    - Terbutaline (Brethine): 0.01 mg/kg SQ, IM q 12 h; or 0.1 to 0.2 mg/kg PO q 12 h
    - Cyproheptadine: 2 mg PO q 12 h (used in cats not responding to the maximum doses of terbutaline and corticosteroids)
- Oxygen therapy

INFORMATION FOR CLIENTS

- The prognosis for cats with asthma is variable.
- If allergens can be determined and exposure decreased before permanent damage occurs, most cats do well.
- Most cats with asthma require periodic medication. Cats with chronic asthma may require continuous medication.
- Aggressive treatment at the veterinary hospital is needed for acute bouts of respiratory distress.
- A cure is usually not possible.

FELINE HEARTWORM DISEASE

Heartworm infection in cats is less common than in dogs (about 5% to 20% of canine prevalence). Clinical symptoms of the disease in cats, however, are often more severe than in the dog, although the worm burden is usually small (Table 12-1). This disease is seen in 38 of the 50 states, mostly along coastal areas and the Mississippi River Valley.

Clinical signs are often different from those seen in dogs. Cough and dyspnea are hallmark signs. The standard ELISA antigen tests are of little value, missing as many as 50% of natural infections. Male cats (age 4 to 6 years) seem predisposed to this condition.

CLINICAL SIGNS

- Cough
- Dyspnea

TABLE 12-1. Feline heartworm disease vs. canine heartworm disease

	DOG	CAT
BIOLOGY OF D. IMMITIS		
Microfilaremia	30%-80% of infected dogs	Rare, transient
Number of adult worms	>50 common	1-3 common
Ectopic migration	Rare	More common
Adult lifespan	Approximately 5 yr	Approximately 2 yr
CLINICAL SIGNS OF HEARTWORM DISEASE		
No signs	Most common	Most common
Respiratory signs	Common	Common
Vomiting	Unusual	Fairly common
Exercise intolerance	Common	Rare
Ascites	Common	Rare
Sudden death	Rare	More common
RADIOGRAPHIC FINDINGS		
Enlarged pulmonary arteries	Characteristic	Characteristic
Blunting/tortuosity	Common	Occasional
Infiltrates in lung	Possible	Possible
Right-sided heart enlargement	Occasional	Rare
Pulmonary artery "knob"	Characteristic	Not seen

- Weight loss, anorexia
- Vomiting
- Lethargy

ACUTE OR PERACUTE PRESENTING SIGNS
- Salivation
- Tachycardia
- Dyspnea
- Hemoptysis, cough
- Central nervous system signs
- Sudden death (uncommon)

DIAGNOSIS
LABORATORY
- Microfilarial tests: Cats are usually microfilaria negative or have too small a number of organisms to be detected.
- Antigen tests: Cats typically have low worm burdens (1 to 2 worms) that are missed by these tests.
- Antibody tests: A negative test is 100% specific; a positive test indicates the following:
    Infection
    Past exposure
    Ectopic infection

RADIOGRAPHY
- Radiographs may show enlarged caudal pulmonary arteries (1.6 times the width of the ninth rib at the ninth intercostal space).

ECHOCARDIOGRAPHY
- An experienced echocardiography technician can detect linear foreign bodies in the pulmonary artery or right ventricle.

TREATMENT
- The use of adulticide in cats is *not recommended* because most infections are self-limiting.

SUPPORTIVE CARE
- Cage rest and confinement
- Cortisone orally to reduce inflammation (see Chapter 2, The Cardiovascular System)

PREVENTION
- Ivermectin (Heartgard, Merial): 0.024 mg/kg PO q 30 days
- Milbemycin: 2000 μg/kg
- Revolution: A monthly spot-on preparation

INFORMATION FOR CLIENTS
- This is a self-limiting disease in cats (elimination of most adult worms occurs within 1 to 2 years).
- Both outdoor and indoor cats are at risk of infection.
- Cats living in areas where heartworm disease is prevalent should be on monthly prevention.

FELINE VIRAL RESPIRATORY INFECTIONS (FELINE VIRAL RHINOTRACHEITIS, CALICIVIRUS)

Even though vaccines are readily available, feline respiratory diseases caused by viral agents continue to be a problem in house cats, in multicat facilities, and in feral cats. The two viral agents responsible for most respiratory problems are feline herpesvirus (FVR) and feline calicivirus (FCV).

FELINE HERPESVIRUS (FELINE VIRAL RHINOTRACHEITIS)

FVR is a highly contagious upper respiratory disease of cats with a high morbidity and moderate mortality and may be extremely severe in young kittens. Infections occur year round in both vaccinated and unvaccinated cats, with clinical symptoms being more severe in the unvaccinated population. Transmission of the virus is via aerosolization (sneezing) and by direct cat-to-cat contact. Queens may transmit the disease to their kittens during grooming. The virus is not hardy and is usually inactivated in the environment within 18 to 24 hours. Cats usually shed the virus for up to three weeks after infection; food dishes, clothing, bedding, and toys can act as fomites for spread of the disease.

CLINICAL SIGNS
- Acute onset of sneezing
- Conjunctivitis (usually severe), purulent rhinitis
- Fever
- Depression
- Anorexia
- Ulcerated nasal planum

- Excessive salivation
- Abortion in pregnant queens
- Corneal ulcers

DIAGNOSIS

- Clinical signs are used most commonly for diagnosis.
- Direct immunofluorescence testing of nasal smears

TREATMENT

SUPPORTIVE THERAPY

- Give fluids (IV, SQ) to correct dehydration.
- Administer broad-spectrum antibiotics.
- Decongestants, vaporization, antihistamines can be administered.
- Nursing care: Clean eyes and nose several times daily.
- Increase the environmental temperature.
- Force-feed or provide a food with a noticeable odor (cats that cannot smell their food tend to not eat). In addition, warming the food may improve the taste to the cat.
- In general, avoid cortisone as an antiinflammatory.
- Decrease stress on the animal.

ANTIVIRAL THERAPY

- Use the following topically for ocular infections:
  Idoxuridine (Stoxil)
  Vidarabine (Vira-A)
  Trifluridine (Viroptic) 1%

PREVENTION

- A good vaccination program prevents this condition.

INFORMATION FOR CLIENTS

- This is a highly contagious disease.
- Vaccinated cats may show mild clinical signs of infection.
- You can transmit this disease to other cats by contact with your hands and clothes.
- Warming food or using an odoriferous type of cat food may improve appetite in sick cats.
- Disinfectants kill FHV-1 viruses.
- This disease is infectious only to cats.

FELINE CALICIVIRUS (FCV)

Like FVR, feline calicivirus infection produces an acute, highly contagious upper respiratory tract disease in the cat. Ulcerative stomatitis is seen frequently with FCV in upper respiratory tract disorders but is not routinely seen with FVR infections. The calicivirus is resistant to disinfectants and can remain active in the environment for several days. The morbidity of the disease is high but mortality low. Clinical signs can appear year round and are most severe in kittens 2 to 6 months of age. Transmission occurs through direct contact with infected cats.

CLINICAL SIGNS
- Fever
- Serous ocular/nasal discharge
- Mild conjunctivitis
- Oral ulcers with increased salivation
- Pneumonia
- Acute arthritis in kittens (limping kitten syndrome)
- Diarrhea

DIAGNOSIS
- Clinical signs
- Viral isolation

TREATMENT
SUPPORTIVE CARE
- Good nursing care
- Broad-spectrum antibiotics
- Force-feed if ulcers prevent cat from eating
- Oxygen therapy (if dyspneic)
- Disinfect environment using bleach

PREVENTION
- A good vaccination program is important.

INFORMATION FOR CLIENTS
- This disease is highly contagious.
- Clinical signs usually last 5 to 7 days.
- Oral ulcers can last 7 to 10 days and require no special treatment.

- Cats that salivate profusely can become dehydrated and may require fluid therapy.
- Force-feeding may be necessary.
- Vaccination is effective in preventing the disease.

PLEURAL EFFUSION

Pleural effusion, the build-up of fluid within the pleural space, results in respiratory distress for the patient. Several diseases are associated with pleural effusion.

Congestive heart failure, especially right-sided failure, represents a principal cause of pleural effusion in both canine and feline patients. As systemic venous hypertension increases, significant amounts of the straw-colored transudate accumulate within the pleural space, resulting in respiratory difficulty.

Any intrathoracic neoplasia can result in pleural effusion through obstruction of lymphatics, inflammation, hemorrhage, or obstruction of venous drainage. It is common to find effusion associated with mediastinal masses (lymphoma), mesotheliomas of the pleura, or metastatic carcinomas. (Primary pulmonary tumors are uncommon in pets.)

Empyema, or purulent exudative pleural effusion, can occur secondary to trauma, foreign body, or pulmonary infection. It can be idiopathic in dogs.

Chylothorax is the condition defined by the accumulation of chylous fluid in the pleural space. *Chyle* is a term used to describe lymphatic fluid arising from the intestine and containing a high concentration of fat. Any disease that elevates systemic venous pressure may result in chylothorax (malignancy, pancreatitis, trauma, infection, parasites, and idiopathic disorders). There is no documented breed or age predisposition for the formation of chylothorax; however, Afghans and oriental breeds of cats seem to have a predisposition to this condition. Older cats are more likely to develop chylothorax than younger cats.

All pleural effusions produce similar clinical symptoms of respiratory distress, dyspnea, cough, and circulatory compromise. Diagnosis is made from physical examination findings, thoracocentesis, cytology, culture and sensitivity, and radiographic findings. See Table 12-2 for a classification of pleural effusions.

CLINICAL SIGNS
- Dyspnea
- May have cough, fever, pleural pain

TABLE 12-2. Guidelines for characterizing effusions other than hemorrhagic

	TRANSUDATE	MODIFIED TRANSUDATE	EXUDATE
Total protein (g/dl)	<2.5	>2.5	>2.5
Nucleated cell count/μl	<1000	<5000	>5000
Horse	<5000	<10,000	>10,000
Predominant nucleated cell type	Mesothelial/ macrophage	Mesothelial/ macrophage	Neutrophil/ macrophage
Horse	Up to 60% may be neutrophils	Up to 60% may be neutrophils	>60% are neutrophils
More common causes	Portal hypertension secondary to liver insuffficiency	Ascites secondary to right-sided cardiac insufficiency	Inflammatory Septic Nonseptic
	Severe hypoalbuminemia	Intestinal disorder (equine)	Intestinal disorder (equine)

From Meyer DJ, Harvey JW: *Veterinary laboratory medicine: interpretation and diagnosis,* ed 2, Philadelphia, 1998, WB Saunders.

DIAGNOSIS

THORACIC RADIOGRAPHS (SIGNS OF PLEURAL EFFUSION)

- Unilateral or bilateral fluid accumulation (usually bilateral) is seen (fluid is visible if there is >50 ml in small animals and >100 ml in large dogs).
- Increased radiopacity is seen on lateral projection in the ventral portion of the thorax with a scalloped appearance due to the presence of fluid between lobes of the lung (Fig. 12-3).
- DV or ventrodorsal (VD) projection shows the following:
  Retraction of lung borders from the thoracic wall
  Blunting of costophrenic angles
  Partial to total obliteration of the cardiac borders
  Widened mediastinum

---

❶ TECH ALERT

Use extreme care when restraining an animal with pleural effusion.

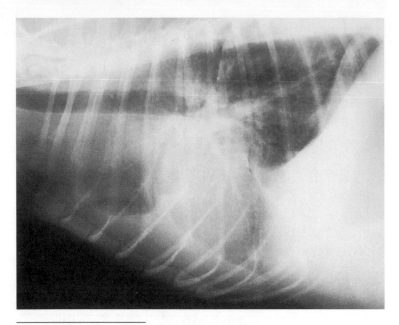

FIGURE 12-3.   Left lateral radiograph of a dog with a large volume of fluid in the pleural space. The cardiac silhouette is partially obscured by surrounding fluid, there are interlobar fissures, and the overall radiopacity of the thorax is increased. In addition, there is an area of radiopacity just dorsal to the sternum, the margins of which are scalloped owing to fluid accumulation in the ventral thorax. (From Thrall DE: *Textbook of veterinary diagnostic radiology,* ed 3, Philadelphia, 1998, WB Saunders.)

THORACOCENTESIS TECHNIQUE
- Prepare and block the skin and the subcutaneous tissues over the seventh or eighth intercostal space, just above the costochondral junction. Use a small needle and 2% lidocaine (Fig. 12-4).
- Insert the chosen device with syringe through the prepared space (a butterfly catheter works well). Avoid the intercostal artery along the caudal portion of the rib.
- Using gentle suction, remove the fluid.
- Send samples to the laboratory for cytology, specific gravity, pH, protein concentration, packed cell volume (PCV), and total and differential white blood cell count (WBC).

TREATMENT
- Treatment depends on the pathology responsible for the effusion.

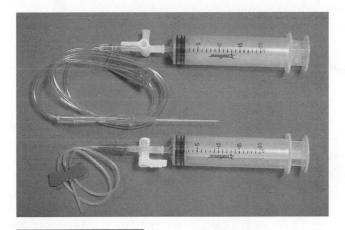

Figure 12-4.   A small-gauge butterfly needle *(bottom)* or an over-the-needle catheter attached to extension tubing *(top)* and a three-way stopcock and syringe are used for needle thoracentesis. (From Fossum TW: *Small animal surgery,* ed 2, St Louis, 2002, Mosby.)

Congestive heart failure

- Treat the underlying disease and use therapeutic thoracocentesis (if needed) to relieve dyspnea.

Neoplasia

- Therapeutic thoracocentesis
- Chemotherapy
- Pleurodesis

Pyothorax

- Tube thoracostomy with continual drainage.
- Antibiotic therapy based on culture and sensitivity results
- Long-term treatment (at least 3 months)
- Good choices for initial treatment include the following:
    Ampicillin: 10 to 20 mg/kg IV, IM, SQ q 6 to 8 h
    Clindamycin: 5 to 10 mg/kg IM, SQ, PO q 12 h
    Chloramphenicol: 45 to 60 mg/kg IM, SQ, IV q 6 to 8 h

INFORMATION FOR CLIENTS

- Whether pleural drainage is required depends on the animal and type of effusion.
- Unless the primary disease is treated, the effusion will return.
- Treatment can be long term and expensive.
- Periodic reevaluation of the patient is required.

Fungal Diseases

Most fungal disease results from the inhalation of fungal spores or from wound contamination. The fungi, found as inhabitants of the animal's environment, damage the host cells by releasing enzymes. They kill, digest, and invade surrounding cells. Some fungi produce toxins. Mycotic diseases are found worldwide but in the United States are endemic along the eastern seaboard, the Great Lakes regions, and the river valleys of the Mississippi, Ohio, and the St. Lawrence waterways (Fig. 12-5).

Inhalation is the common route of infection, and pulmonary symptoms occur with most of the fungal infections. Treatment is often prolonged, and

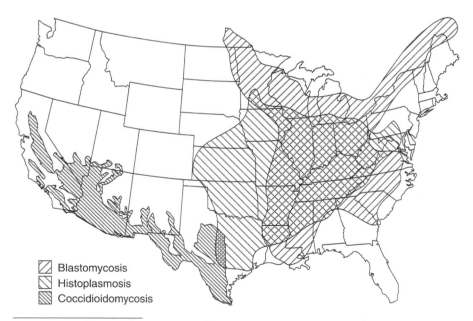

Blastomycosis
Histoplasmosis
Coccidioidomycosis

Figure 12-5. Areas in the United States endemic for blastomycosis, coccidioido-mycosis, and histoplasmosis. (From Ettinger SJ, Feldman EC: *Textbook of veterinary internal medicine,* ed 5, Philadelphia, 2000, WB Saunders.)

relapses are frequent. Fungal infections may disseminate to other organ systems; in these cases the prognosis is usually guarded to grave. Commonly seen fungal diseases of animals include blastomycosis, coccidioidomycosis, histoplasmosis, and aspergillosis.

BLASTOMYCOSIS

Blastomyces dermatitidis is the dimorphic fungus responsible for blastomycosis in the dog and cat. The mycelial phase of the organism is found in soil and cultures but the yeast form is the phase found in the tissues. States having the highest incidence of canine blastomycosis are Kentucky, Illinois, Tennessee, Mississippi, Indiana, Iowa, Ohio, Arkansas, and North Carolina, with some cases occurring in north and south central Texas.

Three clinical forms of the disease exist: primary pulmonary infection, disseminated disease, and local cutaneous infections. Inhalation is the primary route of infection, although wound contamination also occurs. The incubation period is 5 to 12 weeks. The disease is more prevalent in dogs than in cats.

CLINICAL SIGNS
- Anorexia
- Depression
- Weight loss
- Fever (>103° F)
- Cough, dyspnea
- Ocular, nasal discharge
- Wound exudates (serosanguineous to purulent)
- Lymphadenopathy
- CNS signs

DIAGNOSIS

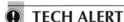 **TECH ALERT**

Lack of appropriate response to antibiotic and corticosteroid therapy should alert the clinician to the possibility of fungal infection.

- CBC and blood chemistry results yield nonspecific signs of chronic disease.
- Hypercalcemia is seen in some dogs.

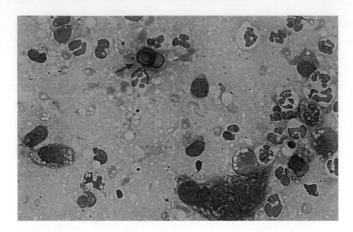

FIGURE 12-6. Pyogranulomatous inflammation from a dog with blastomycosis. A *Blastomyces dermatitidis* organism *(arrow)* is in the center of the field. Neutrophils, macrophages, and an inflammatory giant cell are present. (From Cowell RL, Tyler RD, Meinkoth JH: *Diagnostic cytology and hematology of the dog and cat,* ed 2, St Louis, 1999, Mosby.)

- Cytology: Aspirates or impression smears yield a definitive diagnosis in most cases. The presence of thick-walled budding yeast is typical for *Blastomyces* (Fig. 12-6).
- Radiology reveals generalized diffuse, nodular interstitial pattern. Osseous lesions are seen in the epiphyseal area of long bones.
- Serology testing is available.

TREATMENT
- Amphotericin B is the most effective medication for this disease. It can be administered IV, subconjunctivally, topically, or intraperitoneally. Side effects include anorexia, nausea, vomiting, chills, seizures, fever, anemia, cardiac arrest, and renal impairment.
    - *Slow-drip therapy:* Amphotericin B added to 500 to 1000 ml of 5% dextrose and given over a 3- to 6-hour period (0.09 mg/kg to 0.99 mg/kg 1 to 3 times weekly)
    - *Bolus therapy:* Amphotericin B added to 20 to 50 ml of 5% dextrose and bolused IV (0.09 mg/kg to 0.99 mg/kg 1 to 3 times weekly)
- Ketoconazole: 8.98 mg/kg/day PO for 60 days (33% cure rate)
- Itraconazole: 8.9 mg/kg PO q 24 h (long term)

INFORMATION FOR CLIENTS
- In most cases, blastomycosis is *not* transmitted from animals to humans; however, owners should use caution when handling animals with draining lesions.
- Owners share the same environment as the pet and are likely to be exposed to the same type of fungal spores.
- The prognosis for the pet depends on the stage of the disease and the sex of the pet. Females have a higher survival rate.
- Relapses are common, and treatment may require long-term management.
- The drugs required to treat this disease are expensive.

COCCIDIOIDOMYCOSIS

Coccidioides immitis is a dimorphic soil fungus found in semi-arid areas having sandy soils and mild winters (California, Nevada, Utah, Arizona, New Mexico, and Texas).

Clinical signs of infection may not appear for weeks to years after exposure to the fungal spores. Young, male dogs are most likely to be infected.

CLINICAL SIGNS
- Mild, nonproductive cough
- Low-grade fever
- Anorexia
- Weight loss
- Weakness and depression if systemic
- Lameness, soft tissue swelling, and pain if bone involvement
- Lymphadenopathy may or may not be present
- Myocarditis may or may not be present
- Skin lesions
- Signs of central nervous system involvement

DIAGNOSIS
- CBC/blood chemistry results show nonspecific signs of chronic disease.
- Cytology/biopsy may show thick, double-walled spherical bodies (Fig. 12-7).
- Radiology shows a wide range of parenchymal changes in the lung.
- Serology testing is available.
- Titers greater than 1:16 to 1:32 indicate active disease.

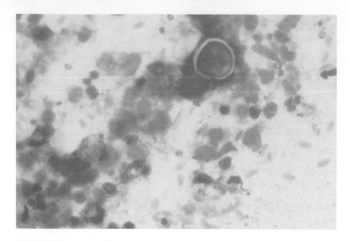

FIGURE 12-7.   Coccidioidomycosis. Large, poorly staining round bodies are the spherules of coccidioidomycosis. (From Baker R, Lumsden JH: *Color atlas of cytology of the dog and cat,* St Louis, 2000, Mosby.)

TREATMENT
- Ketoconazole: 5 to 10 mg/kg PO b.i.d. (dogs)
- Itraconazole: 5 mg/kg PO s.i.d. to b.i.d. (dogs)
- Treatment may be required for 6 to 12 months

INFORMATION FOR CLIENTS
- There is no known risk of animal to human transmission; however, use caution when treating animals with draining lesions.
- Response to treatment usually is good, but relapses are common.
- Life-long treatment may be necessary to keep pet in remission.
- Medications are expensive.

HISTOPLASMOSIS

Histoplasma capsulatum, a dimorphic soil fungus, is endemic in 31 of the 48 continental states (most common in Ohio, Missouri, and the Mississippi River Valley). The fungus has also been associated with bird and bat droppings. Clinical histoplasmosis is as common in cats as in dogs. Inhalation is the prime source of infection with a 12- to 16-day incubation period. The gastrointestinal tract may also be susceptible to *Histoplasma* infection.

CLINICAL SIGNS

FELINE: PULMONARY SIGNS

- Weight loss
- Fever
- Anorexia
- Pale mucous membranes
- May or may not show dyspnea
- Hepatomegaly
- Peripheral lymphadenopathy
- May or may not show ocular lesions

CANINE: GASTROINTESTINAL (GI) SIGNS

- Weight loss
- Diarrhea (large bowel)
- Dyspnea
- Cough
- Pale mucous membranes
- Low-grade fever

DIAGNOSIS

- CBC: Results demonstrate normocytic, normochromic, nonregenerative anemia. Occasionally organisms are seen in neutrophils or monocytes.
- Blood chemistry results are usually normal.
- Cytology/histopathology: Small, round intracellular bodies surrounded by a light halo are seen (Fig. 12-8).
- Radiology: Diffuse or linear pulmonary interstitial patterns (thorax) are seen.
- GI radiographs may indicate ascites.
- Serology is also available (results are often false negative).

TREATMENT

- Ketoconazole: 10 mg/kg PO s.i.d. to b.i.d. for 3 months
- Itraconazole: 5 mg/kg PO s.i.d. to b.i.d. (dogs and cats)

INFORMATION FOR CLIENTS

- Prognosis is fair to good for the pulmonary form, guarded to grave for the systemic form.

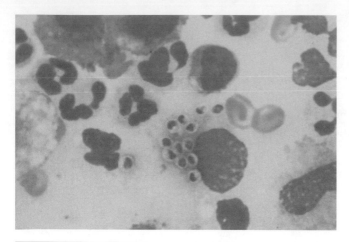

FIGURE 12-8. Histoplasmosis. Mixed inflammatory response surrounding large central macrophage, which contains *Histoplasma* organisms. (From Baker R, Lumsden JH: *Color atlas of cytology of the dog and cat,* St Louis, 2000, Mosby.)

CRYPTOCOCCOSIS

Cryptococcus neoformans is a budding yeast surrounded by a mucoid capsule. Inhalation is the primary means of entry into the body and immunosuppressed animals are more likely to become infected than healthy animals. Organisms commonly grow in avian excreta, especially pigeon droppings.

CLINICAL SIGNS

FELINE (THE MOST COMMON SYSTEMIC MYCOSIS IN THE CAT)
- Nasal cavity and sinus lesions
- Chronic nasal discharge
- Nasal granulomas
- Lymphadenopathy
- May or may not show CNS involvement (seen in 25% of cases)
- Eye lesions (may or may not be seen)
- Low-grade fever, malaise
- Weight loss, anorexia

CANINE (LESS COMMON THAN IN THE CAT)
- Mostly CNS lesions (vestibular dysfunction)
- Skin lesions in about 25% of cases

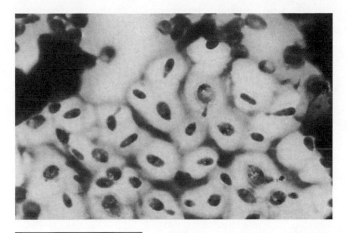

FIGURE 12-9. *Cryptococcus neoformans* is a spherical, yeastlike organism that frequently has a thick, clear-staining mucoid capsule. (From Cowell RL, Tyler RD, Meinkoth JH: *Diagnostic cytology and hematology of the dog and cat,* ed 2, St Louis, 1999, Mosby.)

DIAGNOSIS
- Cytology of aspirates, impression smears, or cerebrospinal fluid (Fig. 12-9)
- Antigen test available commercially

TREATMENT
- Amphotericin B: 0.15 to 0.4 mg/kg IV 3× weekly with 5-Flucytosine
- 5-Flucytosine: 2.75 to 5.5 mg/kg PO q 12 to 24 h
- Ketoconazole: 9.7 mg/kg q 12 to 24 h
- Itraconazole: 9.9 mg/kg PO q 24 h
- Minimum treatment time is 2 months

INFORMATION FOR CLIENTS
- The prognosis is fair to good unless there is CNS involvement, which worsens the prognosis.
- There is no known health hazard to humans.

ASPERGILLOSIS

Aspergillus fumigatus can be found throughout the world in decaying vegetation, sewage sludge, compost piles, and moldy seeds and grains. Inhalation is the most common route of infection, and the nasal cavity is the predominant location of lesions in the dog. Cases of systemic infections have been reported, although they are uncommon.

CLINICAL SIGNS
FELINE ASPERGILLOSIS (UNCOMMON)
- May be immunocompromised with FeLV
- Abnormal lung, GI, liver, spleen, and renal (sometimes) function
- Lethargy, fever
- Weight loss, anorexia

CANINE ASPERGILLOSIS: LOCALIZED INFECTION
- Young to middle age dogs
- Chronic nasal discharge, usually unilateral
- Sneezing
- Stertorous breathing
- Facial pain

CANINE ASPERGILLOSIS: GENERALIZED INFECTION
- Predominantly seen in German Shepherds 1 to 7 years of age
- Weight loss, anorexia
- Fever
- Lameness, back pain, paresis, paralysis
- Ocular signs

DIAGNOSIS
- Radiology shows loss of nasal turbinates, increased lucency, punctate erosions of the frontal bones. Starts unilaterally.
- Biopsy/endoscopy shows yellow-green to gray-black fungal plaques on nasal mucosa. Hyphae are seen on biopsy with hematoxylin and eosin (H&E) stain (Fig. 12-10).

TREATMENT
- Topical clotrimazole: 1 g clotrimazole in 100 ml polyethylene glycol, instilled twice daily through indwelling nasal catheters (surgically placed) or in continuous contact therapy for 1 hour.

INFORMATION FOR CLIENTS
- Localized disease has a fair prognosis, but disseminated disease carries a grave prognosis.

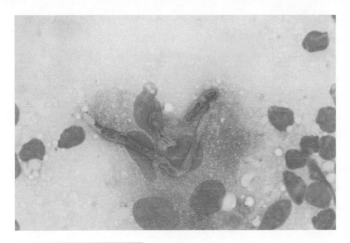

FIGURE 12-10.   Aspergillosis. The long, narrow, angular, negative-stained organism with narrow stained central region is compatible with fungal etiology, probably caused by *Aspergillus* spp. (From Baker R, Lumsden JH: *Color atlas of cytology of the dog and cat,* St Louis, 2000, Mosby.)

- There is no known health risk to humans handling *Aspergillus*-infected animals.
- *Aspergillus* tends to be an opportunistic fungus; infected animals may have a concurrent immune-deficiency problem.

PULMONARY NEOPLASMS

Although primary lung tumors are relatively uncommon in the dog and cat, the lungs can be affected by primary neoplasms, metastatic neoplasms, lymphoma, and neoplasms from surrounding tissues.

The incidence of primary neoplasms in the dog and cat seems to be increasing, although they are still uncommon. Most of the primary tumors seen are adenocarcinomas (70% to 80%), although squamous cell carcinomas, anaplastic carcinomas, fibrosarcomas, osteosarcomas, chondrosarcomas, and benign adenomas are seen occasionally. Pulmonary neoplasms are seen most often in dogs 9 to 12 years old.

Primary tumors may metastasize to regional lymph nodes, long bones, heart, brain, eye, and mediastinal lymph nodes.

Metastatic disease is common in pet animals. Primary tumors involving the thyroid gland and the mammary gland typically metastasize to the lungs, although *any* tumor has the potential to result in metastatic disease.

Although primary lymphoma of the lung has not been reported in pet animals, dogs with multicentric lymphoma frequently have lung involvement.

The prognosis for pulmonary neoplasia depends on the degree of tissue involvement, metastasis of lesions, and lymph node involvement. Surgery is the treatment of choice for tumors that are resectable.

CLINICAL SIGNS
PRIMARY NEOPLASIA
- Cough (usually nonproductive)
- Exercise intolerance
- Weight loss, poor condition
- Dysphagia, vomiting
- Anorexia

METASTATIC NEOPLASMS
- Evidence of a primary tumor at site other than the lung
- All clinical signs as for primary tumor
- Any signs associated with the organ system involved with the primary tumor

DIAGNOSIS
THORACIC RADIOGRAPHS
- Thoracic radiographs do not provide a *definitive* diagnosis—lesions of abscesses, parasitic disease, fungal infections, and bacterial infections may look similar radiographically.
- Radiographs may miss lesions <5 mm in size.
- Two lateral views should be taken (a left and right); to confirm diagnosis, more than one radiologist should read the films.

BIOPSY/CYTOLOGY
- Biopsy and cytology can be performed transthoracically, transbronchially, or surgically.
- Histology provides the *definitive* diagnosis.
- Ultrasound or fluoroscopic guided biopsy can be performed; however, the chances for complications increase (nonrepresentative sample, hemothorax/pneumothorax).

TREATMENT
- Surgical excision is the treatment of choice.
- Lobectomy is usually required for solitary tumors.

- Chemotherapy may reduce the size and effect of the lesion but may not result in increased survival time.

Metastatic tumors
- Surgical removal of the primary tumor is required.
- Chemotherapy should be based on the sensitivity of the primary tumor (although metastatic tumors may have sensitivities different from those of the primary tumor).
- Many tumors are untreatable by the time they are diagnosed.

INFORMATION FOR CLIENTS
- The prognosis for these animals is guarded to grave.
- By the time these tumors are diagnosed they are usually in advanced stages.
- Chemotherapy may help to reduce clinical symptoms produced by the tumor.

thirteen
DISEASES OF THE URINARY SYSTEM

Anatomically, the urinary system is composed of the *kidneys, ureters, bladder,* and *urethra* (Fig. 13-1). The main job of the urinary system is waste removal, although it is also instrumental in red blood cell production, the regulation of water and electrolyte balances, and control of blood pressure. The system is a blood plasma balancer. It processes blood plasma by adjusting the water and electrolyte content, removes waste materials not needed by the body, and returns those necessary substances to the systemic circulation. It also regulates the pH of the plasma. The final product is urine, which is stored for elimination.

The kidneys are located in the retroperitoneal space along the vertebral column from T13–L3. Internally the kidney is divided structurally into the *cortex* (the outer region) and the *medulla* (the inner region) (Fig. 13-2). The "filtration units," or *glomeruli*, are concentrated in the cortical region, whereas the "concentration/exchange tubules," or *nephron loops,* are found in the medulla (Fig. 13-3). Blood enters the kidney and is filtered through the capillaries of the glomerulus. The nephron loop concentrates the filtrate and reabsorbs vital nutrients. The *urine* passes into the ureters and then on to the bladder for storage before elimination.

Clinical disease can result when any portion of this system fails to function properly. The most commonly seen clinical problems involving the urinary system include cystitis, cystic calculi, urinary obstruction, acute and chronic renal failure, and incontinence.

323

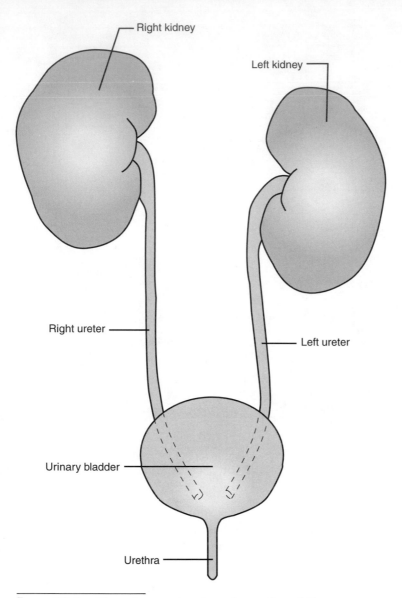

FIGURE 13-1.   The urinary system is made up of two kidneys, two ureters, one urinary bladder, and one urethra. (From Colville T, Bassert JM: *Clinical anatomy and physiology for veterinary technicians,* St Louis, 2002, Mosby.)

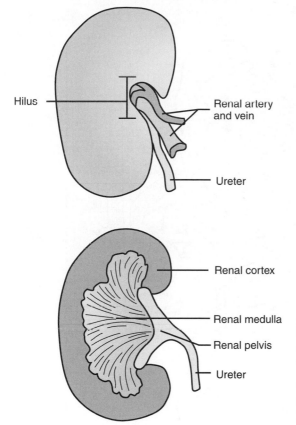

FIGURE 13-2. Frontal section of right kidney. (From Colville T, Bassert JM: *Clinical anatomy and physiology for veterinary technicians,* St Louis, 2002, Mosby.)

CYSTITIS

FELINE CYSTITIS (IDIOPATHIC [INTERSTITIAL] CYSTITIS)

This nonmalignant inflammatory condition, previously known as *feline urologic syndrome* or *feline lower urinary tract disease,* occurs frequently in cats. In a study at The Ohio State University of 132 cats examined for symptoms of irritative voiding (dysuria, hematuria, and pollakiuria), 61% were found to have idiopathic cystitis. The etiology for this disease is unknown, although a virus may be the causative agent. The disease seems to be self-limiting in most cats, with clinical signs subsiding within a week to 10 days. *Any* treatment seems to help because of the self-limiting nature of the cystitis.

Cats with undocumented bacteriuria should not be treated with antibiotics. Needless antibiotic treatment only results in an increased number of antibiotic-resistant organisms.

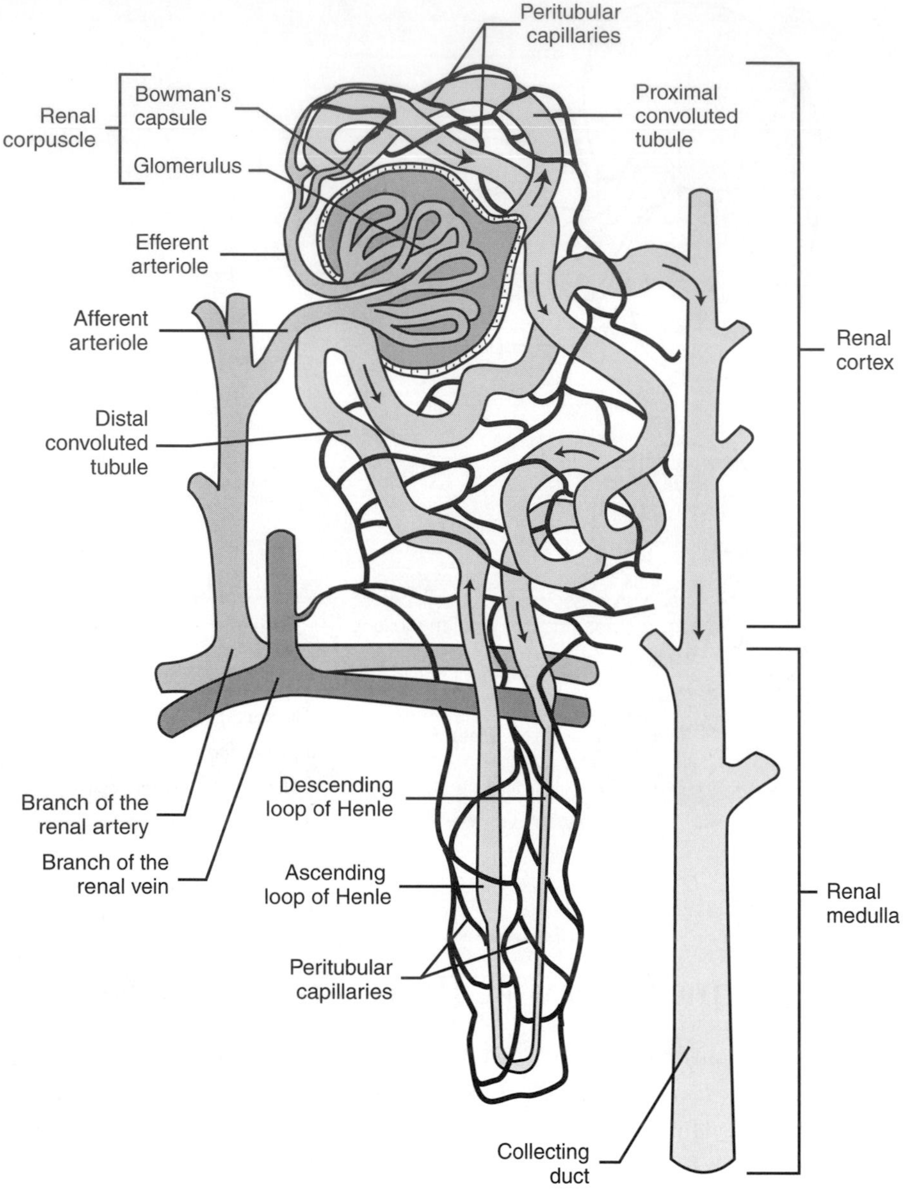

FIGURE 13-3. Fluid flow through the nephron. (From Colville T, Bassert JM: *Clinical anatomy and physiology for veterinary technicians,* St Louis, 2002, Mosby.)

Change of diet may be the most beneficial treatment, especially if it results in dilute urine without an increase in urine pH. If possible, cats should be fed canned food or have water added to their dry food.

Cats should be given places to hide; toys and scratching poles allow cats to exercise normal play behavior and reduce stress, which has been shown to help in the treatment of this disorder.

Use of amitriptyline is advocated to reduce pain and decrease clinical symptoms. A dose just sufficient to calm the cat (2.5 to 12.5 mg/cat) is given orally once daily at bedtime. Monitor liver enzymes while the cat is on this medication.

CLINICAL SIGNS
- Hematuria (frank blood or a pink-colored urine)
- Dysuria (pain on urination)
- Inappropriate urination (e.g., floors, sinks, bathtub)
- More frequent urination (small volumes)

DIAGNOSIS
- Urinalysis: Both dipstick and sediment examination should be performed to rule out bacterial cause or systemic disease.
- Urine culture is negative.
- Radiographic contrast studies may indicate irregular mucosal lining and thickened bladder wall, or radiographs may be normal.

TREATMENT
- Avoid unnecessary use of antibiotics unless urinalysis indicates a bacterial cause.
- Change diet to produce a dilute urine.
- Provide amitriptyline to relieve clinical signs and ease discomfort (2.5 to 12.5 mg/cat PO at bedtime).
- Antiinflammatory medications should be used with caution. (There have been *no* positive clinical effects seen in controlled studies.)
- Administer propantheline 7.5 mg PO q 72 h to relieve incontinence until the condition resolves.

INFORMATION FOR CLIENTS
- This disease is self-limiting.
- This may be a recurring problem.
- There is no definitive cure.

- Reduction of stress in the cat's environment helps prevent recurrence.
- It may be difficult to change the diet. Be creative and patient.

CANINE CYSTITIS (BACTERIAL CYSTITIS)

Although bacterial urinary tract infection accounts for only 1% to 3% of all feline cystitis, it is the most common cause of cystitis in the dog.

The urinary tract is normally sterile (free of bacteria) and resistant to infection. Natural defense mechanisms such as frequent voiding of urine, urethral and ureteral peristalsis, glycosaminoglycans in the surface mucosal layer, pH, and constituents of the urine assist in preventing the invasion of bacteria into lower urinary tract structures.

Urinary tract infections are most commonly the result of ascending migration of bacteria up the urethra. The blood-borne route does not seem of much importance in animal infections. The motility of some bacteria such as *Escherichia coli* and *Proteus* spp. may assist in this migration. Once in the bladder, the microorganisms must adhere and colonize the mucosal lining. Bacteria that may be nonpathogenic in the normal animal may be virulent in hosts with altered immunity.

CLINICAL SIGNS

- Increased frequency of urination
- Hematuria
- Dysuria
- Cloudy urine, abnormal odor
- Frequent licking of the urethral area

DIAGNOSIS

- Urinalysis: Dipstick and sediment examination show increased white blood cell count (WBCs) and bacteria.
- Urine culture and sensitivity: Collect by cystocentesis and culture within 30 minutes for best results. This should *always* be done.

TREATMENT
PREVENTION

- Avoid unnecessary use of indwelling urinary catheters.
- Use a closed system when using indwelling urinary catheters (Fig. 13-4).
- Avoid trauma to the urinary tract during surgical procedures.

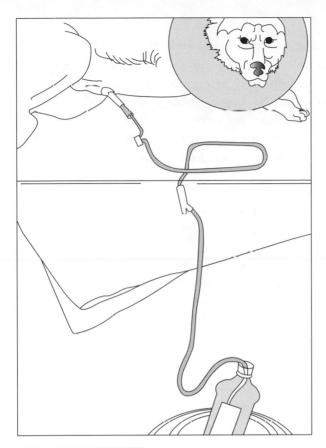

FIGURE 13-4. Collection apparatus in place for continuous urine drainage. Note that collection container is below the level of animal's urinary bladder.

ANTIBIOTICS
- Choice should be based on culture and sensitivity results.
- Empiric choice of antibiotics: drug should attain effective concentrations in the urine and tissue. Some good choices include the following:
    Ampicillin: 11 mg/kg PO q 8 h
    Amoxicillin trihydrate (clavulanate potassium): 10 to 20 mg/kg PO q 8 h
    Trimethoprim-sulfonamide: 15 mg/kg PO q 12 h
    Cephalexin: 30 to 40 mg/kg PO q 8 to 12 h
    Enrofloxacin: 2.5 to 5 mg/kg PO q 12 h

> ❗ **TECH ALERT**
>
> Treatment recommendations include the following:
> - Select the least expensive, least toxic, most effective antibiotic to start treatment. Because of frequency of urination, it is recommended to dose the drug every 8 hours when possible. Treatment should be of sufficient duration to eliminate the bacteria.
> - Treatment for acute infections should be for 10 to 14 days. Chronic or relapsing infections require 4 to 6 weeks of treatment.

INFORMATION FOR CLIENTS
- Most uncomplicated urinary tract infections resolve without treatment.
- If antibiotics are needed, make sure you give them as directed and for the prescribed time period to avoid creating resistance to the drug.
- Relapses are common (many relapses are due to inadequate treatment).
- The prostate may be the source of recurring infections in males.
- Repeat cultures during treatment to follow progress.

FELINE UROLITHS AND URETHRAL PLUGS

A detailed description of feline uroliths is beyond the scope of this text. Students are referred to veterinary medical texts for more information.

"Plugged" cats are a frequent occurrence in the small animal hospital. The inability to pass urine may have serious and even fatal consequences. Two common causes of urethral obstruction in the cat are uroliths and urethral plugs. These terms should not be used synonymously because they are physically distinct from one another. *Uroliths* are polycrystalline concretions comprised of minerals with a small amount of matrix. *Urethral plugs* consist of small amounts of minerals in a large amount of matrix. This section discusses each of these as they affect urinary tract disease in the cat.

FELINE UROLITHS

A number of different minerals can be found in feline uroliths (Fig 13-5). These include the following:
- Struvite (approximately 60%)
- Calcium oxalate (27%)
- Ammonium urate (5.5%)

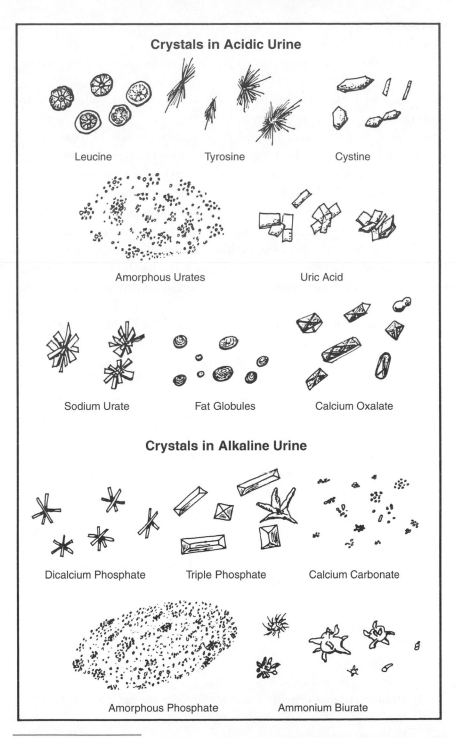

FIGURE 13-5.   Various types of crystals that may be found in urine. (From Pratt PW: *Laboratory procedures for veterinary technicians,* ed 3, St Louis, 1997, Mosby.)

- Cystine
- Mixed mineral

Uroliths, also called *bladder stones,* may be located anywhere in the urinary tract. Some are radiopaque and are easily diagnosed by radiographs (e.g., calcium oxalate, urates, and struvites), whereas others are radiolucent and require double-contrast cystography to be seen.

In most cases, the cause of urolith formation cannot be determined, although studies show that diets high in magnesium produce struvite uroliths experimentally in cats. Obese, older cats (>2 years) seem to be predisposed to urolith formation. There seems to be no breed predisposition for struvite uroliths; however, Burmese, Himalayan, and Persian breeds have a higher prevalence of calcium oxalate uroliths. Cats that form uroliths typically have concentrated urine with altered pH (either too alkaline or too acidic). Cats with uroliths may be asymptomatic or may present with signs of lower urinary tract disease or urethral obstruction. Spontaneous reabsorption of uroliths has been documented.

Uroliths that remain in the bladder can damage the bladder lining, resulting in secondary bacterial infections and hematuria. Small uroliths that become lodged in the outflow tract present a special problem. As urine flow out of the bladder stops, the bladder distends with urine. This results in a back up of urine through the ureter and into the kidney, virtually halting renal filtration and urine production. The cat becomes azotemic within 24 hours, and clinical signs relating to this begin to be evident at this time. If the obstruction to urine flow is not relieved within 3 to 6 days, the cat will die.

This section focuses on struvite uroliths because they are the most commonly seen type. Please refer to medical texts for treatment of other types of uroliths.

CLINICAL SIGNS
- Signs depend on the degree of trauma and whether urinary obstruction is present.
- Some cats with bladder or renal uroliths may be asymptomatic. However, clinical signs include the following:
    Hematuria
    Dysuria
    Urinating in strange places
    Straining to pass urine (owners may report the cat is constipated)
    Vomiting
    Collapse, death

DIAGNOSIS
- Radiology may show uroliths on routine films.
- If there is a strong suspicion, a double contrast study should be done.
- Ultrasonography locates the position of uroliths in the urinary tract.
- An analysis of the uroliths is critical for proper treatment.
- Small uroliths may be collected by catheter while obtaining a urine sample.

MEDICAL TREATMENT
- Struvite uroliths can be treated by inducing their dissolution. By feeding a diet that reduces urine pH to 6 to 6.3 and that is low in magnesium (Prescription Diet Feline S/D), uroliths will dissolve. This type of diet may also prevent the recurrence of these uroliths.
- Dissolution is usually completed in 4 to 8 weeks. Animals should be examined radiographically every 2 to 4 weeks to monitor the dissolution process. Continue the diet for 1 month after all uroliths have disappeared.
- Antibiotic treatment helps prevent secondary bacterial infections that may occur in traumatized tissues.

SURGICAL TREATMENT
- Consider surgery for uroliths that fail to resolve with diet.
- Postsurgical radiographs should be taken to ensure that all uroliths have been removed.

TREATMENT (FOR OBSTRUCTIVE UROLITHS)
MEDICAL TREATMENT
- Uroliths must be retrograded back into the bladder or removed from the urethra. Using a well-lubricated, open-end feline catheter, which has been atraumatically inserted in the urethra (under sterile technique), and a saline or lactated Ringer's solution, gently propulse the urolith back toward the bladder. This reestablishes urine flow and allows time for further medical management (Fig. 13-6).
- Dietary dissolution: Diets low in magnesium, which promote a urine pH of 6 to 6.3, are recommended for dissolution of struvite uroliths (Prescription Diet Feline S/D). Dissolution may take 4 to 8 weeks. Follow progress with radiographs taken every 2 to 4 weeks. Continue diet for 1 month after uroliths disappear from the radiographs.
- Antibiotics should be used to prevent secondary bacterial infections in

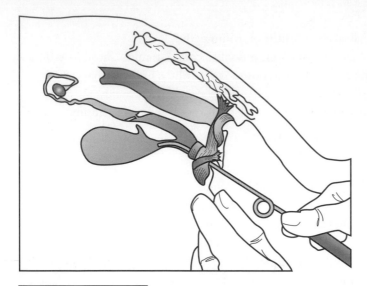

Figure 13-6.   Introducing a urethral catheter into a female cat.

the already traumatized urinary tract. Choice may be empirical or based on culture and sensitivity results.

- Monitor the animal's urine flow daily, because reobstruction may occur.

Surgical treatment
- Surgery (perineal urethrostomy with or without cystotomy) should be performed if uroliths cannot be removed from the urethra or dissolution does not occur. Owners should be advised of the risks associated with perineal urethrostomies (increased bladder infections, strictures). A cystotomy may be needed to remove the uroliths in the bladder.

INFORMATION FOR CLIENTS
- If the uroliths do not dissolve, surgery is required.
- Feed the cat the prescription diet exclusively. No treats or table food!
- Medical treatment requires periodic monitoring by radiography and urinalysis.
- Canned food provides more dietary water and, hence, more dilute urine.
- Antibiotics may be needed long term in certain cats.
- Long-term effects from a perineal urethrostomy may include a higher susceptibility to bacterial cystitis and strictures.

- Your veterinarian should examine cats that seem "constipated" as soon as possible.

FELINE URETHRAL PLUGS

The same factors associated with the formation of uroliths are risk factors identified in urethral plug formation in the cat. Plugs contain varying quantities of minerals in proportion to large amounts of matrix. The matrix is a muco-protein associated with a local host defense mechanism in the urinary tract. Plugs may also contain red blood cells, white blood cells, epithelial cells, bacteria, and spermatozoa.

CLINICAL SIGNS

- Straining to urinate; cat may be crying or just spending excessive time in the litterbox (seen more frequently in male cats)
- Vomiting
- Dehydration
- Collapse (subsequent death within 3 to 6 days)

DIAGNOSIS

- Diagnosis is the same as for other causes of urethral obstruction.
- Bladder is enlarged and firm on palpation.
- There is a history of straining or no urine production.
- Radiographs reveal enlarged bladder.
- Serum chemistries demonstrate elevations in BUN, creatinine, potassium, phosphate, and calcium. (Levels measured depend on length of time urine flow has been obstructed.)

TREATMENT

❶ TECH ALERT
Reestablish urethral patency!

- Manual restraint alone or in combination with anesthetics may be used. Propofol, isoflurane, or short-acting barbiturates may be used.

❶ TECH ALERT
If anesthetic drugs are used, remember that doses *less* than those recommended are required in azotemic cats.

- Step-wise attempt to relieve the obstruction is recommended:

    Gently massage the urethra, using the thumb and forefinger, to break up the plug. (This technique is rarely successful.)

    Gently attempt to compress the bladder to force the plug out of the urethra. (This technique almost never works when used alone.)

⓿ TECH ALERT

Exercise caution with these techniques. You can easily rupture a distended bladder.

Cystocentesis, when properly performed, reduces the back pressure on the plug in the urethra, allowing it to be hydropulsed into the bladder. Cystocentesis also provides the technician with a sample suitable for urinalysis and culture and sensitivity.

- Back-flush the urethra with sterile saline or lactated Ringer's solution.
- Periodically reevaluate the patency of the urethra because reobstruction may occur.
- *Avoid the use of indwelling catheters because they further traumatize the bladder and urethra and provide an introductory route for ascending bacterial infections.* If these must be used, make sure that you use a soft, nontraumatic catheter that is connected to a closed, sterile drainage system (see Fig. 13-4).
- Surgery: Perineal urethrostomy may be attempted if the obstruction cannot be removed.

UROLITHIASIS (CANINE)

There appears to be a small incidence of this problem in the dog. Several studies indicate a prevalence of less than 1%. In the dog, the most common type of urolith is composed of magnesium ammonium phosphate, whereas calcium oxalate, urate, cystine, and calcium phosphate uroliths occur less frequently (see Fig. 13-5).

Uroliths form from urine supersaturated with specific substances (minerals). Many researchers think that minerals precipitate from the urine after formation of a crystal nidus or center. Once the nidus has formed, mineral continues to be deposited around it forming a "stone" or urolith. This process may be complete in as little as a few days to as long as several weeks.

After formation, uroliths may pass out of the urinary tract, continue to grow in the tract, dissolve, or become inactive. The sequelae of those that remain within the urinary tract can include dysuria, infection, partial or complete obstruction, and polyp formation.

Urinary tract infection is common in dogs with urolithiasis. Uroliths mechanically disrupt the mucosal lining of the tract, opening it to bacterial colonization and partially disrupting bladder emptying. Small uroliths can become lodged in the penile urethra of the male, and slightly larger ones can block the female urethra. Complete obstruction to urine outflow can quickly result in destruction of renal parenchyma and uremia.

COMMON TYPES OF CANINE UROLITHS

STRUVITE (MAGNESIUM AMMONIUM PHOSPHATE)

No specific breed predilection for this type of urolith has been demonstrated; however, approximately 80% of dogs with struvite uroliths are females between the ages of 3 and 8 years. Alkaline urine, urease producing bacteria, and dietary minerals facilitate the formation of this type of urolith.

Treatment includes long-term antibiotics (until radiographs demonstrate absence of uroliths); urine acidification using dietary management (Hill's Prescription Diet S/D); and dietary restriction of urea, phosphorus, and magnesium (S/D diet). Use of the prescription S/D diet results in the dissolution of struvite uroliths within approximately 1 to 3 months. Dietary modification and long-term use of prophylactic antibiotics can prevent recurrence.

CALCIUM OXALATE

This type occurs primarily in male dogs between the ages of 5 and 12 years. Veterinarians are seeing an increase in the number of cases involving this type of urolith because of the frequent use of medical protocols to dissolve struvite, urate, and cystine uroliths. The increased rate of oxalate uroliths may also be related to diets high in animal protein.

Hypercalcemia is a significant finding in dogs with calcium oxalate uroliths. Studies of dogs that develop calcium oxalate crystals also show the presence of a structural abnormality in the urine protein *nephrocalcin*, which is necessary for inhibition of calcium oxalate crystal growth.

At present, surgical removal is the only means of removing calcium oxalate uroliths. Prevention should be aimed at reducing serum calcium levels, reducing dietary calcium and oxalate (milk products), and restricting dietary sodium. Diets such as Hill's Prescription U/D, which are moderately protein restricted (and low in calcium, sodium, and oxalate), are available. Other choices include Hill's Prescription Canine W/D and K/D diets.

URATES (AMMONIUM URATES AND OTHERS)

Uric acid is one of several biological products of purine nucleotide metabolism. Ammonium urate is a salt of this acid and accounts for most of the purine uroliths in the dog.

Dalmatian dogs are predisposed to urate uroliths. The hepatic and renal metabolic pathways in this breed result in a secretion of excess uric acid from the kidneys (2 to 4 times that found in non-Dalmatian breeds). This excess predisposes the breed to urate uroliths. Other breeds with an increased incidence include the English Bulldog, Miniature Schnauzer, Shih Tzus, and Yorkshire Terriers. Most of the dogs affected are males between the ages of 3 and 6 years. Research suggests that prolonged use of severely restricted protein diets in non-Dalmatian dogs may be responsible for urate urolith formation.

Treatment includes use of dietary management to dissolve the uroliths (Hill's Prescription Diet U/D), allopurinol (15 mg/kg q 12 h) to decrease uric acid production, alkalinization of the urine with sodium bicarbonate or potassium citrate (pH = 7.0), and control of concurrent bacterial infection in the urinary tract.

CLINICAL SIGNS (STRUVITE UROLITHS)
- Dysuria
- Hematuria

DIAGNOSIS
- Urinalysis will show crystalluria, hematuria, increased protein, and increased numbers of bacteria.
- Radiographs can be used to verify the number, location, and size of uroliths. Double-contrast studies can be used to visualize some uroliths (urates). Radiographs may miss uroliths <3 mm in size.
- Serum chemistry may indicate metabolic abnormalities underlying urolith formation.
- Stone analysis is important for formulating treatment plans; commercial laboratories are available for stone analysis, or one can "guesstimate" the stone type based on several criteria (Table 13-1).

TABLE 13-1.   Predicting mineral composition of uroliths

PREDICTORS

MINERAL TYPE	URINE pH	CRYSTAL APPEARANCE	URINE CULTURE	RADIOGRAPHIC DENSITY	RADIOGRAPHIC CONTOUR	SERUM ABNORMALITIES	BREED PREDISPOSITION	SEX PREDISPOSITION	COMMON AGES
Magnesium ammonium phosphate	Neutral to alkaline	Four- to six-sided colorless prisms	Urease-producing bacteria (*Staphylococcus*, *Proteus*, *Enterococcus*, *Mycoplasma*)	+ to ++++	Smooth, round, or faceted; may assume shape of bladder or urethra	None	Miniature Schnauzer, Bichon Frisé, Cocker Spaniel	Females (>80%)	2-8 yr or younger
Calcium oxalate	Acid to neutral	Dihydrate salt, colorless envelope or octahedral shape; monohydrate salt-spindles or dumbbell shape	Negative	++ to ++++	Rough or spiculated (dihydrate salt); small, smooth, round (monohydrate salt); sometimes jackstone	Occasional hypercalcemia	Miniature Schnauzer, Lhasa Apso, Yorkshire Terrier, Miniature Poodle, Shih Tzu, Bichon Frisé	Males (>70%)	5-12 yr

From Ettinger SJ, Feldman EC: *Textbok of veterinary internal medicine,* ed 5, Philadelphia, 2000, WB Saunders.
+, Low radiographic density; ++, moderate radiographic density; ++++, high radiographic density (opaque); −, radiolucent (not visible).

Continued

TABLE 13-1. Predicting mineral composition of uroliths—cont'd

PREDICTORS

MINERAL TYPE	URINE pH	CRYSTAL APPEARANCE	URINE CULTURE	RADIOGRAPHIC DENSITY	RADIOGRAPHIC CONTOUR	SERUM ABNORMALITIES	BREED PREDISPOSITION	SEX PREDISPOSITION	COMMON AGES
Urate	Acid to neutral	Yellow-brown amorphous shapes or sphericals (ammonium urate)	Negative	− to ++	Smooth, round, or oval	Low urea nitrogen and serum albumin in dogs with hepatic portal systemic shunts	Dalmatian, English Bulldog, Miniature Schnauzer, Yorkshire Terrier	Males (>85%)	1-4 yr
Calcium phosphate	Alkaline to neutral (brushite forms in acidic urine)	Amorphous, or long thin prisms	Negative	++ to ++++	Smooth, round, or faceted	Occasional hypercalcemia	Yorkshire Terrier, Miniature Schnauzer, Cocker Spaniel	Males (>60%)	7-11 yr
Cystine	Acid to neutral	Flat colorless, hexagonal plates	Negative	+ to ++	Smooth to slightly irregular, round to oval	None	English Bulldog, Dachshund, Basset Hound	Males (>90%)	1-8 yr
Silica	Acid to neutral	None observed	Negative	++ to +++	Round center with radial spoke-like projections (jackstone)	None	German Shepherd, Golden Retriever, Labrador Retriever, Miniature Schnauzer	Males (>90%)	9 yr

TREATMENT

MEDICAL

- Treatment must be aimed at decreasing urine saturation, increasing the solubility of crystalline material in the urine, and increasing urine volume:

    Diet change to decrease solids in the urine

    Promote acid urine

    Induce diuresis

- Provide antibiotics for infection.

SURGICAL REMOVAL

- Remove uroliths not manageable with medical treatment or in patients with severe infections.
- The cause of urolith formation must be medically addressed.

NONSURGICAL REMOVAL

- A catheter can be used to remove small uroliths.
- Urohydropulsion, or digital pressure on the bladder of an anesthetized dog, can propulse small stones through the urethra.

INFORMATION FOR CLIENTS

- A special diet may be needed throughout the life of the dog.
- Table scraps and treats should be limited.
- Long-term antibiotics may be necessary to control the urinary tract infection.
- Uroliths may recur at any time.
- Follow-up laboratory tests and radiographs are required to monitor medical dissolution of uroliths.

RENAL FAILURE

Renal failure is one of the most commonly seen diseases in veterinary medicine. The unique structure of the kidney and its job of filtration and waste management within the body predispose the kidney to numerous insults throughout the life of the animal. Approximately 20% of the total cardiac output passes through the kidney at any one time. The content of this blood is filtered through the glomerular capillary membrane, removing small molecules, electrolytes, drugs, and other materials. These substances become the glomerular filtrate, which enters the proximal convoluted tubule, the nephron loop, and the distal convoluted tubule before leaving the kidney by way of the collecting duct, the renal pelvis, and the ureter. The tubules reabsorb water and other substances necessary to maintain bodily functions. Waste materials are excreted. The resulting product, urine, leaves the kidney to be stored in the bladder for elimination from the body. A reduction in blood flow to the nephron (hypoperfusion) or damage to the nephron unit itself can result in renal failure. Renal failure may be *acute* or *chronic*. In both types of failure, the nephron unit is damaged and glomerular filtration declines, resulting in *azotemia*, a build-up of toxins within the body. The azotemia produces the clinical symptoms of renal failure.

ACUTE RENAL FAILURE

Acute renal failure refers to an *abrupt* decrease in glomerular filtration resulting in azotemia. This is usually the result of hypoperfusion or nephrotoxic injury to the kidney, which results in damage to the proximal convoluted tubular cells or those of the ascending nephron loop. Nephrotoxic drugs such as the aminoglycosides (gentamycin, streptomycin, amikacin), cephalosporins (cephalexin, cephalothin), the sulfonamides (Albon, Di-Trim, Primor), chemotherapeutic agents, antifungal medications, some analgesics (acetaminophen), and anesthetics (Metofane) can produce acute renal failure if used for prolonged periods or at high doses. The most common nontherapeutic agents that produce renal damage include ethylene glycol (antifreeze), heavy metals, and hemoglobin. Infections, immune-mediated diseases, and hypercalcemia have also been implicated as causes of acute renal failure in both humans and animals.

Nephrotoxic injury may affect any portion of the nephron; when one section is damaged, the entire unit is lost. Destroyed nephrons cannot be replaced by the body, but other nephron units have the ability to hypertrophy (enlarge) in an attempt to maintain normal renal function. Acute renal failure occurs in three distinct phases: (1) induction—the time from the initial insult until decreased renal function is apparent; (2) maintenance—the period during which renal tubular damage occurs; and (3) recovery—the time during which renal function improves, existing nephrons hypertrophy and compensate for those damaged, and tubular repair occurs (when possible).

Risk factors for acute renal failure include disorders affecting renal perfusion (shock, hypovolemia, hypotension, dehydration), electrolyte (potassium, calcium, sodium) disturbances, administration of nephrotoxic drugs, systemic diseases, and increased age. Technicians should be alert to these risk factors when monitoring patients under anesthesia or with trauma, and in older patients with systemic diseases. Every effort should be made to normalize blood flow through the kidney and avoid prolonged periods of hypotension and/or hypovolemia. Careful monitoring of pulse quality, hydration status, packed cell volume, total solids, and body weight make it possible to observe early changes that may suggest the development of acute renal failure. Early intervention may prevent permanent damage to the kidneys.

Signs of acute renal failure are often nonspecific. Patients may present with a variety of symptoms, but a good history can pinpoint a recent ischemic episode or toxin exposure. The kidneys are enlarged and painful on palpation, and the patient may be exhibiting signs of azotemia such as anorexia, vomiting, diarrhea, and weakness. Laboratory tests indicate an active urine sediment, normal to increased hematocrit, acidosis, and normal to elevated potassium levels. Blood urea nitrogen (BUN) and creatinine levels may be elevated. Patients may be oliguric (passing decreased amounts of urine) or polyuric (passing increased amounts of urine).

Treatment is aimed at restoring renal hemodynamics, relieving any tubular obstruction, discontinuing any potentially nephrotoxic drugs, and promoting cellular repair. Intravenous fluid therapy (with isotonic saline being the initial fluid of choice) is the hallmark of therapy for acute renal failure. Correction of acid-base imbalances and control of hyperphosphatemia, hyperkalemia, and gastroenteritis is also necessary. Although treatment may not restore renal function to previous levels, it will improve the clinical picture, make the animal feel better, and give the kidney time to heal.

The prognosis for acute renal failure in veterinary patients is guarded and is related to the severity of the azotemia. Patients with nephrotoxic injuries have a slightly better prognosis than those with hypoperfusion injury. Older patients have a less favorable prognosis than younger patients.

Great care should be taken to protect patients at risk of developing acute renal failure. With careful monitoring, early recognition, and aggressive therapy, renal damage can be kept to a minimum in many patients.

CLINICAL SIGNS
- Oliguria, polyuria
- Fever (if infectious)
- Kidneys painful on palpation
- Vomiting and diarrhea
- Anorexia
- Dehydration

DIAGNOSIS

- Physical examination
- History of ischemic episode or toxin exposure
- Urinalysis-active sediment, casts
- Blood chemistries: increased packed cell volume (PCV), elevated BUN and creatinine, elevated potassium, phosphorus, acidosis

TREATMENT

- Intravenous fluid therapy: Initial choice is isotonic saline
- Discontinue potentially nephrotoxic drugs
- Intestinal protectants:
  Metoclopramide: 0.2 to 0.5 mg/kg IV, IM, PO q 6 to 8 h
  Cimetidine: 2.5 to 5 mg/kg IV q 8 to 12 h
  Sucralfate: 0.05 to 1 g PO q 6 to 8 h
- Phosphate binders if necessary: Maalox, Amphojel
- Sodium bicarbonate: BW (in kg) $\times 0.3 \times (20 - T_{CO_2}) = $ mEq. Give one half IV slowly over 15 to 30 minutes.
- Diuretics:
  Dopamine: 1 to 5 µg/kg/min IV
  Furosemide: 2 to 6 mg/kg IV q 8 h
  Mannitol (20%): 0.5 to 1.0 g/kg IV slowly over 15 to 20 minutes

INFORMATION FOR CLIENTS

- Although renal function may be improved with treatment, it may never return to completely normal levels.
- The prognosis for this disease is guarded.
- The underlying condition responsible for the acute renal failure may require long-term management.
- Care must be taken to avoid events that would precipitate further damage to the kidneys. Appropriate diet and water access must be assured for these pets.

Chronic Renal Failure (CRF)

Chronic renal failure is a common disease of older pets. It represents an irreversible and progressive decline in renal function due to destruction of the nephron units. The course of the disease may be months to years with clinical signs appearing when nephron loss reaches levels that result in the development of azotemia. The incidence of disease is higher in older animals (dogs >8 years, cats >10 years), but it can be seen in animals of any age. CRF may be congenital, familial, or acquired in origin. Cats seem to be more affected than dogs, with an increased frequency of disease seen in Maine Coon, Abyssinian, Siamese, Russian Blue, and Burmese breeds. Whatever the cause, the irreversible destruction of the nephron results in uremia and its related clinical symptoms.

One of the most frequently seen signs of uremia is gastrointestinal upset—anorexia, weight loss, vomiting, diarrhea, constipation, and stomatitis (oral ulceration). Unfortunately, owners do not often associate these signs with renal disease, and pets go undiagnosed until symptoms become severe.

As the kidneys lose their ability to concentrate urine, signs of polydipsia, polyuria, and nocturia may develop. This loss of concentrating ability is the result of impairment of ADH response, disruption of the countercurrent mechanism and renal tubular epithelium, along with the increased solute load passing through the remaining nephrons.

Other signs of CRF include arterial hypertension, nervous system dysfunction (dullness, lethargy, tremors, seizures), scleral injection, retinal lesions, and acute blindness. An increased tendency for bruising may also be seen. Most animals with moderate to advanced CRF are anemic due to a decreased level of the hormone erythropoietin, which is produced by the kidney. The severity and progression of the anemia correlate well with the degree of renal failure.

Metabolic imbalances also produce hyperphosphatemia (decreased excretion), hypokalemia (increased secretion; especially in cats), proteinuria, and metabolic acidosis.

Therapy should be individualized based on the patient's needs. Owners should be informed that the loss of renal function is permanent and progressive. The prognosis for CRF is poor. Treatment is aimed at correcting metabolic imbalances and minimizing clinical symptoms. General goals of treatment are to decrease the dietary protein intake while maintaining adequate caloric intake, provide relief of nausea and vomiting through the use of H_2-receptor antagonists like cimetidine or ranitidine, correct the hypokalemia with oral potassium therapy, and avoid dehydration by giving SQ or IV fluids. Phosphorous binding agents such as Amphojel can be used to control hyperphosphatemia.

In cases in which systemic hypertension is compromising kidney function, therapy with ACE inhibitors (enalapril), β-adrenergic antagonists (propranolol), or calcium channel blockers (diltiazem) may improve renal function. Loop diuretics (furosemide) may be used to reduce blood pressure by reducing body fluid loads.

Epoetin (Epogen), a replacement erythropoietin, may be given to correct the anemia. Some clinicians have suggested using calcitriol to decrease parathyroid hormone levels and thereby normalize calcium and phosphorus balance, but studies indicate that the risks of using calcitriol outweigh the benefits, and its use is no longer suggested in CRF.

It should be stressed to owners that all these treatments only *limit or slow* the progression of this disease. The condition is fatal.

CLINICAL SIGNS
- Dullness, lethargy
- Weakness
- Weight loss
- Anorexia
- Vomiting and/or diarrhea (constipation in cats)
- Polyuria/polydipsia
- Gait disturbances: Cervical ventriflexion in cats
- Sudden blindness

DIAGNOSIS
- Acidosis
- Anemia
- Increases in BUN, creatinine
- Hyperphosphatemia
- Hypercalcemia or hypocalcemia
- Hypokalemia
- Proteinuria

TREATMENT
- Treatment should be aimed at supportive care and correction of imbalances (dehydration, electrolytes, metabolic acidosis, gastrointestinal symptoms).
- Provide fluids IV or SQ for dehydration: Suggested fluids include a mixture of two parts D_5W and one part lactated Ringer's solution (by volume) supplemented with potassium as needed. Owners can be instructed in how to give SQ fluids at home (two to three times weekly or as needed to maintain hydration).
- Potassium gluconate (Tumil-K or Kaon Elixir): 2 to 6 mEq/cat/day
- Phosphorous binders: Aluminum hydroxide (Amphojel) 30 to 90 mg/kg PO s.i.d. to t.i.d. with meals

- Calcium carbonate (for hypocalcemia): 100 mg/ kg/day PO
- Sodium bicarbonate: 8 to 12 mg/kg q 8 to 12 h. (A solution can be prepared that contains 80 mg/ml by adding one third of an 8-ounce box of sodium bicarbonate to 1 quart of water.) Store in the refrigerator, and give 1 to 1.5 ml/4.5 kg of body weight.
- Cimetidine: 5 to 10 mg/kg PO, IM, IV t.i.d. to q.i.d.
- Ranitidine: 1 to 2 mg/kg PO b.i.d.
- Sucralfate: 0.5 to 1 tablet (dogs); 0.25 to 0.5 tablet PO q 8 h (cats)
- ACE inhibitors
  Enalapril: 0.25 to 3.0 mg/kg PO q 12 to 24 h
- Calcium channel blockers
  Diltiazem: 0.5 to 1.5 mg/kg PO q 8 to12 h (dogs); 1.0 to 2.25 mg/kg PO q 8 to 12 h (cats)
- β-adrenergic antagonist
  Propranolol: 2.5 to 10 mg PO b.i.d. to t.i.d. (dogs); 2.5 to 5 mg PO b.i.d. to t.i.d. (cats)
- Diuretics
  Furosemide: 0.5 to 2 mg/kg PO q 8 to 12 h
- Hormones
  Epoetin: 50 to 150 U/kg SQ 3 times weekly
- Calcitriol: 1.5 to 3.5 ng/kg/day PO (use is no longer recommended; see text)
- Vitamin B supplements

Diets lower in protein and sodium have been suggested to slow the progression of CRF; however, studies have shown no protective benefit from diets low in protein. If the BUN values are above 75 mg/dl, then protein restriction is suggested to reduce nonrenal toxicities.

INFORMATION FOR CLIENTS
- This is a progressive, irreversible disease.
- Treatment is aimed at *slowing* the progression and relieving clinical symptoms.
- Treatment with SQ fluids at home is required to maintain the pet's hydration. You will be instructed in how to give the fluids.
- You can improve the palatability of renal diets by warming foods and adding tasty liquids such as tuna oil, clam juice, or broth. You should limit foods containing high levels of salt.
- Eventually your pet will experience a decrease in its quality of life. You may have to consider euthanasia.

URINARY INCONTINENCE

Urinary incontinence is frequently reported by clients, especially when older pets are involved. Urinary incontinence can be defined as the loss of voluntary control of micturition. It occurs for a variety of reasons, and treatment should be based on an accurate diagnosis. In the dog and cat, urethral closure is not accomplished by a single anatomic sphincter, but is primarily the result of smooth muscle tone along the entire urethra in female dogs and along the proximal fourth of the urethra in males. When the urethral closure pressure is greater than the bladder pressure, urine remains stored in the bladder until voluntary urination occurs. When bladder pressure rises above urethral closure pressure, incontinence occurs. Other types of incontinence include neurogenic incontinence, nonneurogenic incontinence, paradoxical incontinence, and miscellaneous incontinence.

Neurogenic incontinence may be seen in animals with spinal cord disease or trauma. Intervertebral disc disease, vertebral fractures, inflammation, or neoplasia of the spinal cord can disrupt normal neural function to this region of the urinary system, resulting in a paralytic bladder. In these animals the bladder overdistends with urine, increasing intravesical urine pressure and resulting in dribbling of urine.

Nonneurogenic causes of incontinence include congenital abnormalities such as ectopic ureters, patient urachus (seen in younger animals), endocrine imbalances following ovariohysterectomy (estrogen deficiency), urethral sphincter mechanism (degenerative changes, urinary surgery), and hypercontractile bladder.

Paradoxical incontinence occurs in patients with partial obstruction of the urethra. This situation is encountered most frequently in male dogs. The bladder becomes overdistended with urine, which cannot pass because of some type of obstruction, raising the intravesical pressure above that of the urethra and resulting in incontinence.

Miscellaneous causes can include primary diseases of the bladder, which result in replacement of normal bladder wall smooth muscle tissue with fibrous or neoplastic tissue. Classification of urinary incontinence is shown in Table 13-2.

CLINICAL SIGNS
- Owner reports urine leakage when the pet is sleeping or exercising.
- Perineal area of pet is always wet.
- Signs of concurrent urinary tract disease are present.

TABLE 13-2.   Classification of urinary incontinence

TYPE	NORMAL MICTURITION	INVOLUNTARY DRIBBLING OF URINE	OVERDISTENDED BLADDER	SMALL, CONTRACTED BLADDER	ABILITY TO CATHETERIZE BLADDER
Neurogenic	Absent	Present	Present	Absent	Easy
Nonneurogenic	Present	Present	Absent	Absent	Easy
Paradoxical	Absent	Present	Present	Absent	Difficult
Miscellaneous	Absent	Present	Absent	Present	Variable

From Osborne CA, Low DG, Finco DR: *Canine and feline urology,* Philadelphia, 1972, WB Saunders.

- Older spayed female dogs and noncastrated male dogs are predisposed to this condition.

DIAGNOSIS
- Urinalysis
- Radiology/cystography
- Serum chemistries to rule out polyuria from endocrine disease

TREATMENT
- Treatment should be based on determination of a specific etiology.

ENDOCRINE IMBALANCE IN SPAYED FEMALE DOGS
- Diethylstilbestrol (DES): 0.1 to 1 mg/day PO for 3 to 5 days, then 1 mg/week PO

URETHRAL SPHINCTER HYPOTONUS
- Phenylpropanolamine (Propagest, Reed & Carnick): 12.5 to 50 mg PO q 8 h

🚯 **TECH ALERT**

Avoid use of phenylpropanolamine in patients with glaucoma, hypertension, diabetes mellitus, and prostatic hypertrophy.

HYPERCONTRACTILE BLADDER
- Propantheline (Pro-Banthine, Roberts): 7.5 to 30 mg PO q 8 to 12 h (dogs); 5 to 7.5 mg PO q 24 to 72 h (cats)
- Oxybutynin (Ditropan): 0.5 to 1 mg PO q 8 to 12 h (small dogs, cats); 1.25 to 3.75 mg PO q 12 h (large dogs)

🚯 **TECH ALERT**

Side effects from anticholinergic medications include sedation, ileus, vomiting, constipation, dry mouth, dry eyes, and tachycardia. Their use is contraindicated in patients with glaucoma.

INFORMATION FOR CLIENTS
- A complete physical and laboratory work-up is needed to diagnose the specific cause of your pet's incontinence.

- Medication doses may need to be adjusted to achieve success in stopping the incontinence.
- Drugs used to treat incontinence cannot be used in pets having other health problems such as glaucoma, diabetes mellitus, hyperthyroidism, or cardiac disease.
- If the incontinence is due to trauma or inflammation, it may correct itself with time.
- If the incontinence is due to paralytic bladder, you may need to catheterize your pet several times daily or manually express the bladder to prevent overfilling.

BIBLIOGRAPHY

Baker R, Lumsden JH: *Color atlas of cytology of the dog and cat,* St Louis, 2000, Mosby.

Birchard SJ, Sherding RG: *Saunders manual of small animal practice,* ed 2, Philadelphia, 2000, WB Saunders.

Bojrab JM, editor: *Current techniques in small animal surgery,* ed 4, Baltimore, 1998, Williams & Wilkins.

Bonagura J, editor: *Kirk's current veterinary therapy XIII,* Philadelphia, 2000, WB Saunders.

Brinker WO, Piermattei DL, Flo GL: *Handbook of small animal orthopedics and fracture treatment,* Philadelphia, 1983, WB Saunders.

Case LP et al: *Canine and feline nutrition,* ed 2, St Louis, 2001, Mosby.

Colville T, Bassert JM: *Clinical anatomy and physiology for veterinary technicians,* St Louis, 2002, Mosby.

Compendium of veterinary products, Port Huron, MI, 1991, North American Compendiums.

Cowell RL, Tyler RD, Meinkoth JH: *Diagnostic cytology and hematology of the dog and cat,* ed 2, St Louis, 1999, Mosby.

Crow SE, Walshaw SO: *Manual of clinical procedures in the dog, cat, and rabbit,* ed 2, Philadelphia, Lippincott-Raven Publishers.

DeLahunta A: *Veterinary neuroanatomy and clinical neurology,* ed 2, Philadelphia, 1983, WB Saunders.

Dunn J: *Textbook of small animal medicine,* Philadelphia, 1999, WB Saunders.

Edwards NJ: *Bolton's handbook of canine and feline electrocardiography,* ed 2, Philadelphia, 1987, WB Saunders.

Edwards NJ: *ECG manual for the veterinary technician,* Philadelphia, 1993, WB Saunders.

Ettinger SJ, Feldman EC: *Textbook of veterinary internal medicine,* ed 5, Philadelphia, 2000, WB Saunders.

Ettinger SJ, Suter PF: *Canine cardiology,* Philadelphia, 1970, WB Saunders.

Fossum TW: *Small animal surgery,* ed 2, St Louis, 2002, Mosby.

Greene CE: *Infectious diseases of the dog and cat,* ed 2, Philadelphia, 1998, WB Saunders.

Han CM, Hurd CD: *Practical diagnostic imaging for the veterinary technician,* ed 2, St Louis, 2000, Mosby.

Hendrix CM: *Diagnostic veterinary parasitology,* ed 2, St Louis, 1998, Mosby.

Holmstrom SE: *Veterinary dentistry for the technician and office staff,* Philadelphia, 2000, WB Saunders.

Holmstrom SE, Frost P, Eisner ER: *Veterinary dental techniques for the small animal practitioner,* ed 2, Philadelphia, 1998, WB Saunders.

Kesel L: *Veterinary dentistry for the small animal technician,* Ames, 2000, Iowa State University Press.

Kirk RW, editor: *Current veterinary therapy IX: small animal practice,* Philadelphia, 1995, WB Saunders.

Kittleson MD, Kienle RD: *Small animal cardiovascular medicine,* St Louis, 1999, Mosby.

La Croix NC, van der Woerdt A, Olivero DK: Nonhealing corneal ulcers in cats: 29 cases (1991-1999), *J Am Vet Med Assoc* 218(5):733, 2001.

Lavin LM: *Radiography in veterinary technology,* ed 2, Philadelphia, 1991, WB Saunders.

McCurnin DM, Bassert JM: *Clinical textbook for veterinary technicians*, ed 5, St Louis, 2002, WB Saunders.

Meyer DJ, Harvey JW: *Veterinary laboratory medicine,* ed 2, Philadelphia, 1998, WB Saunders.

Nelson RW, Couto CG: *Small animal internal medicine,* ed 2, St Louis, 1998, Mosby.

Olmstead ML: *Small animal orthopedics,* St Louis, 1995, Mosby.

Osborn CA, Low DG, Finco DR: *Canine and feline urology,* Philadelphia, 1972, WB Saunders.

Pederson NC et al: Feline immunodeficiency virus infection, *Vet Immunol Immunopath* 21:111, 1989.

Plumb D: *Veterinary drug handbook,* ed 3, Ames, 1999, Iowa State University Press.

Pratt PW, editor: *Laboratory procedures for veterinary technicians,* ed 4, St Louis, 1997, Mosby.

Pratt PW, editor: *Principles and practice of veterinary technology,* St Louis, 1998, Mosby.

Ralston S, Stemme K, Guerroro J: *Preventing heartworm disease in cats,* Proceedings of an Innovations Session (Merck), 1997, North American Veterinary Conference.

Scott DW, Miller WH Jr, Griffin CE: *Muller and Kirk's small animal dermatology,* ed 6, Philadelphia, 2001, WB Saunders.

Slatter D: *Fundamentals of veterinary ophthalmology,* ed 3, Philadelphia, 2001, WB Saunders.

Sodikoff CH: *Laboratory profiles of small animal diseases: a guide to laboratory diagnosis,* ed 3, St Louis, 2001, Mosby.

Thibodeau GA, Patton KT: *Anatomy and physiology*, ed 3, St Louis, 1996, Mosby.

Thrall DE: *Textbook of veterinary diagnostic radiology,* ed 4, Philadelphia, 2002, WB Saunders.

Tortora GJ, Grabowski SR: *Principles of anatomy and physiology,* ed 9, New York, 2000, John Wiley & Sons.

Wyman M: *Manual of small animal ophthalmology,* New York, 1986, Churchill Livingstone.

Zoonosis updates from the Journal of the American Veterinary Medical Association, ed 2, Schaumburg, IL, 1995, American Veterinary Medical Association.

Index

A

Page numbers followed by f indicate figures; t, tables;
b, boxes.